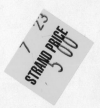

Primer for the Nonmedical Psychotherapist

Primer for the Nonmedical Psychotherapist

Joyce A. Bockar, M.D.

S P Books Division of
SPECTRUM PUBLICATIONS, INC.
New York

Distributed by Halsted Press
A Division of John Wiley & Sons

New York   Toronto   London   Sydney

Spectrum Publications, Inc.
86-19 Sancho Street, Holliswood, N.Y. 11423

Distributed solely by the Halsted Press Division of John Wiley & Sons, Inc. New York.

Fifth Printing

Library of Congress Cataloging in Publication Data

Bockar, Joyce A
   Primer for the nonmedical psychotherapist.

   Includes index.
   1. Psychopharmacology. 2. Drug abuse.
3. Psychological manifestations of general diseases
I. Title.
RC483.B62   616.8'91   75-41476
ISBN 0-470-15230-3

Printed in the United States

Preface

This book is written with the belief that nonmedical psychotherapists will and should be doing the vast majority of psychotherapy in the near future. The need for counseling or psychotherapy is steadily increasing in our fast-changing society. The number
of psychiatrists cannot keep pace with this increasing demand for
psychological services, to which the increasing number of nonmedical practitioners attests. Additionally, it seems a phenomenal
waste of medical training for M.D.s to engage exclusively in psychotherapy. On the other hand, it is of the utmost importance that
people who think themselves in need of psychotherapy be given a
thorough medical screening before embarking on their treatment,
to insure that they do not have a medical, surgical or neurological
disease which is appearing as a psychological difficulty. It is with
the knowledge that it is unlikely that the hundreds of patients
coming to nonmedical therapists will have received this medical
screening that this book was written. It is with the hope and belief
that nonmedical practitioners, given a little of what I call "medical
intelligence," which is in essence, a high index of suspicion, will be
able to detect those signs which indicate that they should send the
patient to an M.D. for further investigation. The difference
between a psychiatrist and all other nonmedical practitioners of

psychotherapy is that his medical training, both consciously and unconsciously, alerts him to cues that the patient often gives, that some medical disease may be in process which may be responsible for the psychological complaints.

Furthermore and most important, the psychiatrist knows what questions to ask so as to eliminate or decrease the suspicion of the medical possibilities which cross his mind. Albeit, most of the diseases which could be confused with psychological illness are uncommon, or downright, rare. However, it is truly a tragedy when medical disease of this nature is missed, and the patient spends a great deal of time, effort and money with no relief of his sympotomatology through psychotherapy. In the first section of this book, chapters are devoted to describing the most common psychological syndromes seen in the everyday practice of psychotherapy. They are coupled with descriptions of certain medical diseases, most of which, although uncommon, are curable by medical or surgical intervention. The types of questions which an M.D. might ask the patient are included with each description so that the nonmedical practitioner can try to eliminate the probability of that specific illness, much the way an M.D. would do so. Naturally all questions which could give medical cues cannot be included nor does the first section attempt to make the nonmedical practitioner an M.D. What it does do, hopefully, is raise the index of suspicion of the lay professional so that he can "sniff out" possibilities that should alert him to get the patient to an M.D. A very commonly encountered psychiatric disease, i.e., schizophrenia, is not included in the description of common practice entities because very few if any medical diseases per se mimic this entity. The effects of certain drugs and some organic psychoses, however, do mimic schizophrenia and these are included under organic psychoses. This is not intended to be a textbook of psychiatry, therefore some familiarity with psychological disease states is assumed, and a full description and classification of schizophrenia is beyond the scope of this volume.

The second section of this book is devoted to giving the lay professional specific knowledge of drugs, both prescription and illicit, that are most commonly used by patients with whom he comes in contact. Many of these drugs are prescribed by the referring, consulting or supervising M.D. with which most lay professionals are associated. It is written with the realization that often the prescribing M.D. rarely sees the patient again for long intervals. The lay professional is often left, therefore, in a considerable quandry, not knowing if new symptoms are side effects of the prescribed drugs, or how to deal with the very frequent patient complaints about dosage, timing or mixture with other drugs or alcohol.

Certain drugs have proven in study after study, that they are more effective than psychotherapy alone (see phenothiazines). It is the author's opinion that drugs plus psychotherapy are more effective than either alone and that drugs to relieve anxiety and depression should be used in almost every case where significant syndromes of that nature exist. Giving the nonmedical practitioner familiarity with these medications will hopefully increase the likelihood that he will see these drugs as an adjunct to his practice. Furthermore, it will give him enough knowledge to be able to suggest to his "backup" M.D. which class of drugs he thinks his patient should be prescribed. It will hopefully enable him to distinguish certain side effects from psychological symptoms. Most importantly it will enable him to know when to send the patient back to the prescribing M.D. for a re-evaluation of the medication or its dosage. Also included in the second section are several of the illicit drugs now in increasingly common usage among younger patients, and several of the abused prescription drugs such as barbiturates and amphetamines whose abuse continues by all generations. Since no drug is more abused than alcohol a separate chapter on alcohol and alcoholic syndromes has been included. By including descriptions of effects, addiction syndromes and withdrawal syndromes, the lay professional is in a more knowledgeable position to decide when and if his patient needs hospitalization for these problems.

In summary, this book is dedicated to the patient and to his protection. It is written with the realization that, increasingly in the present and surely in the future, the vast burden of patients in need of counseling or psychotherapy will be handled by psychologists, social workers, lay analysts, psychiatric nurses, chaplains, paramedical personnel and truly lay indigenous workers. It is written with the spirit that the more these lay professionals know about possible medical illness in their patients, and the more they know about prescription and illicit drugs, the more likely it is that the patient will receive the best medical and psychological care.

Contents

Primer for the Nonmedical Psychotherapist

CHAPTER I

Anxiety . . . Or?

There is a network of nerves in the body called the sympathetic nervous system.* This system is responsible for the physical signs that are associated with acute and sometimes chronic anxiety. The sympathetic nervous system is important in maintaining the integral functioning of the many organ systems in the body. One of the functions of the sympathetic nervous system is to prepare the person for "fight or flight." This function is very important, because anxiety is the subjective experience that accompanies the body's preparation to run away from danger, or stay there and fight it. If the body is going to run or fight, more blood has to go to the muscles, which means, since there is only a limited supply of

*The sympathetic nervous system is really a division of the body's whole nervous system. This division, however, acts often as a whole, and has two common chemicals, one of which mediates the transmission of the final nerve impulse to the receptor nerve cell and both of which are secreted by the adrenal glands in time of stress. These chemicals are norepinephrine and epinephrine and are discussed in the final chapter.

1

blood, that it must come from other places. It does. The sympathetic nerves to the intestines cause them to temporarily slow down or stop digestive processes—the familiar "knot" in the stomach. This stopping of the digestive process allows the blood supplying that process to be diverted. Since the body is preparing for possible injury, the blood vessels to the skin constrict, shifting the blood to more vital internal organs and thus insuring that less bleeding will occur from cuts. The released epinephrine from the adrenal glands goes to the lungs and opens up the bronchi (breathing tubes) to allow more oxygen-containing air in faster. The sympathetic nerves to the heart increase its rate, so the increased oxygen will be pumped to the muscles faster. The pupils dilate, teleologically presumably to be better able to see the danger. Putting all this together, we can now have a picture of the patient experiencing or complaining about anxiety attacks.

The patient will state that he gets cold (blood vessels to skin shut down), he begins to sweat, he feels his heart beating rapidly, he feels shaky and tremulous and his stomach may feel cramped. He may feel nauseous and he may feel the urge to vomit, urinate or defecate. (That's where the expression for anxiety "I could have shit in my pants" probably comes from.) The patient may also complain of feeling light-headed or dizzy, which may be derived from excessive breathing, i.e., hyperventilation, which we will take up shortly. This describes an anxiety "attack," but many people have chronic anxiety and exhibit one or more of the components of the attack almost constantly. They may complain that their hands and feet are always cold; that they have to urinate very frequently; that their stomach is constantly upset or "'in a knot" or that they are frequently dizzy and confused.

Subjective anxiety entails the following conditions: skin cold, sweaty, pupils dilated, hands have a fine, fast tremor (shaking), heart beat is rapid, breathing rapid, digestion slowed, tendency to nausea or vomiting, to defecation or to diarrhea. Remember these signs, since in certain instances if *one* is changed, it may mean medical illness. Furthermore, these signs will serve as a reference for many drug effects, and some withdrawal syndromes, as well as some medical illnesses.

Below is an example of a medical illness, namely hyperthyroidism, which, *from the patient's verbal report*, mimics anxiety in almost all the respects mentioned except *one*.

HYPERTHYROIDISM

Hyperthyroidism is not an uncommon disease. It is caused by overactivity of the thyroid gland, which is located at the base of the neck in front of the larynx. In this disease the patient may complain of feeling anxious, he will be sweaty, he may have a fine tremor of his hands, his heartbeat and breathing are rapid, he tends to have diarrhea. He has all the symptoms of anxiety already discussed—except one. Cold! Hyperthyroid patients are *hot*! Their skin is warm to the touch and they may in fact have an elevated body temperature. Hyperthyroid patients have additional symptoms, which distinguish them from patients with anxiety, if one remembers to ask. They generally have an increased appetite, but even in the face of *increased food intake*, they generally *lose weight*. One of the cardinal questions for this disease, as well as a host of other medical and psychological diseases, is "Have you lost or gained weight recently?, and if so, how much and in how long a span of time?" Ten pounds per year is a significant loss or gain. The hair texture of hyperthyroid patients often tends to become finer or thinner. A frequent accompaniment of hyperthyroidism is protrusion of the eyeballs, so that the person looks like his eyes are too far out of the sockets. One must observe carefully however for black people of certain African origins have naturally protruding eyeballs, and this is merely a racial characteristic.

In short, the person with hyperthyroidism strongly resembles the person with a sympathetic reaction except for the following: (1) they are hot-sweaty not cold-sweaty, (2) they are losing weight or maintaining weight even in the face of increased appetite and increased food intake (no other disease except untreated diabetes, which does not have the associated sympathetic activity, causes *weight loss* with *increased* appetite), and (3) they are constantly in the "anxiety attack" state, whereas the anxious patient is usually not.

Ask the person who is complaining of symptoms that sound like a sympathetic reaction whether he is hot when he is sweaty or cold when he is sweaty. If he thinks he is hot when this reaction is going on or even if he says he is cold or doesn't know, ask further about weight loss and appetite, hair thinning, and if he is continuously in this state (with rapid heartbeat, subjective anxiety and possibly shaking). As a rough guide, a weight loss *without* dieting of ten pounds in one month should cause immediate medical referral. If *any* of his answers are cause for question you can suggest he have his thyroid checked by an M.D.

In all fairness to everyone, obviously not everyone who is *chronically* anxious exhibits necessarily *any* of the signs of *acute* anxiety. Someone chronically anxious may or may not have persistently cold feet or a "knot" in their stomach. The point is that very often patients complain of these symptoms and are quite frightened by them—especially those involved in hyperventilation. It is comforting in these cases, to both the therapist and the patient, to ascertain that these symptoms are most likely due to anxiety. However, if atypical symptoms develop, it should cause referral to an M.D.

HYPERVENTILATION

Along with their anxiety attacks, many patients tend to hyperventilate—that is, breathe too fast and too deeply for too long. This tends to deplete their body of carbon dioxide which is extremely important in maintaining the pH of body fluids and the form that certain dissolved salts take in the blood. (pH is a measure of acidity.) Suffice it to say that when somebody hyperventilates the balance of calcium salts in the blood is changed. When this balance is changed, numbness and tingling (paresthesias) of the fingertips, hands, and feet and occasionally of parts further up the extremities may ensue. (Paresthesias also occur when your foot "falls asleep", but for an entirely different reason.) The hyperventilation also causes light-headedness, dizziness, and often pains in the chest, peculiarly enough, around the heart. The patient rarely tells you he is overbreathing. Instead, he complains of numbness and tingling of the extremities, chest or heart pain, light-headedness, etc. He may or may not relate these occurrences to subjective anxiety, and it is highly unlikely he would relate them to specific environmental precipitants. All these symptoms, including the chest pain, disappear spontaneously soon after he stops hyperventilating, and calms down, even if he never realized he was either anxious or hyperventilating.

There are several medical diseases which have many symptoms

in common with the hyperventilation syndrome. People who have chronic kidney disease are often irritable, depressed, anxious, chronically nauseous as well as constipated, and may present themselves to the nonmedical practitioner before seeing an M.D. for therapy for depression or generalized increase in anxiety and irritability. Interestingly enough, a derangement in their calcium metabolism also induces numbness and tingling of the extremities, but this generally does not subside as easily as when these symptoms are related to hyperventilation. Be highly suspicious and refer immediately to a doctor, anyone who complains of constant paresthesias of the extremities.

It is really quite interesting that there is a great difference in probable disease entities if the patient complains of numbness and tingling in *one* hand or *one* foot alone. In general, the paresthesias from hyperventilation are most often symmetrical. However, parethesias starting in the left *or right* armpit or shoulder and radiating down either arm can signify anything from compression of a nerve root in the neck, to temporarily insufficient blood supply to the heart causing chest pain (angina pectoris), to an actual heart attack, if accompanied by severe pain or crushing sensation in the chest. Here it is necessary to consider the age and sex of the patient, the frequency, duration, and recurrence of attacks, all of which contribute to determining the likelihood of any of the above problems. In general, hyperventilation is thought to occur somewhat more frequently in younger women, but I have seen a case or two in teenage boys. Heart attacks are rather rare in women before the menopause. A man of 45 or older, however, with his *first* attack of anxiety, profuse sweating, chest pain, and paresthesias of the left or right arm should be immediately suspected of having a heart attack *in progress*, and be seen as an emergency in a hospital or doctor's office. Regardless of sex, if the patient is over 50 with *recurrent* attacks of anxiety and chest pain around the heart, with or without paresthesia, he should be seen by a doctor for further evaluation of what may turn out to be angina pectoris. (A note about age here. Men under 45 and women smokers under 45 are getting heart attacks at an increasing rate. It is wise to refer all patients with symptoms of angina pectoris or with first attacks of the type described above to an M.D.)

To review for a moment, then, the typical patient with anxiety attacks accompanied by hyperventilation is likely to be female, between 12 and 40 years of age. Her attacks may be accompanied by chest pain, symmetrical paresthesias, and light-headedness, all of which disappear rapidly when the attack is over. Nerve root compression, angina pectoris, and heart attacks do not have pain which readily subsides without medical treatment. The paresthesias of these problems are generally not symmetrical and the chest pain is of much greater intensity. If your patient is less than 45 all three possibilities are less likely. First attacks in either sex over 35 should be suspect, but more so for men. If the symptoms have been occurring for a while before the patient sought therapy, occur variably during the day, are recognized by the patient as having some relationship to subjective anxiety, and most important, disappear spontaneously and rapidly (within 30-60 minutes) then it is most likely that the patient has hyperventilation syndrome. I had a patient like this who was 26, female and swore she was having a heart attack when it occurred. A mild tranquilizer prevented the attacks or aborted them in every instance. This would be *rarely* true in angina, highly unlikely in nerve root compression, and impossible if a true heart attack were in progress. Although attacks of angina pectoris are accompanied by anxiety and can subside spontaneously, angina pectoris mostly occurs in men over 35 and women usually beyond the menopause.

One further note on this subject. Most patients with hyperventilation syndrome will probably have consulted a doctor about their symptoms. Unfortunately, I have had several patients with this syndrome tell me that the doctor said it was *nothing*, and told them to see a psychiatrist. Patients have a hard time believing that dizziness or light-headedness, chest pain and paresthesias are "nothing," or worse, "psychosomatic." I have found it very helpful to explain to the patient that she is experiencing real symptoms, but that these are due to overbreathing even if she doesn't realize it. You can tell her that she can prove this to herself by ending the symptoms herself, simply by breathing in and out of a paper bag. That's right. If she holds the bag loosely over her face and breathes into it and out of it for a period of time—usually five or ten minutes—she can stop the symptoms. Really the best way to do this is to put the bag over her head and tell her to breathe normally in it. But you need quite a relationship with a patient before you can put a paper bag over her head!

HYPOGLYCEMIA

There is another syndrome which although it is quite rare, is indistinguishable from recurrent full-blown anxiety attacks, unless you ask some very specific questions. Even then, only certain blood tests can definitely make the diagnosis. This syndrome is the often discussed and debated hypoglycemia (hypo- low, glycemia-blood sugar).

There are several well published M.D.s who do not believe that this syndrome is at all rare, and tend to blame a host of psychological ailments on it. The large weight of medical opinion, however, supports the contention that it is truly rare in its pure form. The reason that it is indistinguishable from a sympathetic reaction, is because when blood sugar falls too low the body responds with a sympathetic reaction.

People who really suffer from this disorder may have attacks of inexplicable anxiety and consult a nonmedical therapist. If you ask them what times during the day they have those anxiety attacks, they are likely to state that they wake up with them. This is because their blood sugar, like everyone elses, is lowest in the morning, the time separated by the most hours from a mealtime. A very astute patient may have already learned that as soon as he has his orange juice and sweet roll, the symptoms subside. Unfortunately, most patients don't make that connection. If you question closely, you may find that he gets "anxiety" attacks at 11:00 A.M. (before lunch), about two or three hours after lunch, before dinner, and about two or three hours after dinner. Human beings are such that we try to make events that happen seem rational to us. So the patient may have some very plausible reasons for his distress, particularly if he's been in therapy for a while and has become somewhat more psychologically oriented. There is really no sure-fire way to judge, because even if the patient wakes up with his head pounding, cold and sweaty and shaking, he may still have anxiety—either from dreaming or from having to face an anxiety-producing day. If the symptoms occur *every* morning and *every* day two or three hours after meals (despite the fact that you or the patient feel that he is terrified of a man he sees just before his coffee break), then it is worth checking with an M.D. One further way to determine whether the patient is anxious or hypoglycemic is to tell him to eat sugar in some form (e.g., donut or candy bar) when he feels these "anxiety" attacks coming on. If this completely relieves the symptoms within ten minutes to a half hour, he may indeed have hypoglycemia. If, on the other hand, probably due to the mere suggestion of the therapist, he feels either instantaneous relief or relief only after one hour or more, it is very doubtful that he has hypoglycemia. However, it is certainly worth having him take the diagnostic tests, if the patient has persistent recurrent anxiety attacks, occurring at a fairly specific time of day, especially in the morning before breakfast, which are unabated by psychotherapy or tranquilizers for a period greater than two months. (A word about relief by tranquilizers. Although it is possible for tranquilizers to temporarily relieve most of the symptoms, in true hypoglycemia complete relief can only be obtained by eating some form of sugar.) Be suspicious, but remember hypoglycemia is rare.

POSTCONCUSSION SYNDROME

Subjective anxiety, irritability, increased sensitivity to noise, light, heat or other environmental stimuli, fatigability, insomnia, headaches, and difficulty in concentrating can all be due to psychological disturbances. They can also be the results of a head injury whether mild or severe, with or without unconsciousness accompanying the injury. It is always necessary, therefore, to ask a new patient whether he has had a head injury or whiplash injury within the last year or two, because the most common presenting symptom of this syndrome is *anxiety.*

It is impossible to separate out the psychological reactions to a head injury from those due to injury to the brain itself. Sometimes the accident triggers off a whole neurotic reaction, in which many of the above symptoms are present. The longer the time between the accident and the initiation of symptoms the more likely it is that you are dealing with neurotic symptoms and not the direct results of brain injury.

Persistent headaches which are aggravated by changes in posture, such as stooping or bending over, point to changes due to brain injury. Memory loss for incidents one to two hours before the injury is common if consciousness was lost. Amnesia for periods of years prior to the injury is exceedingly rare and should be suspected of being hysterical (not medical).

Frequently the anxiety and other symptoms do not appear for one to two weeks after a minor injury and the patient may not make the connection between a minor accident and his sudden development of symptoms. It is always wise if a history of head injury or whiplash is obtained to refer the patient to an M.D. before continuing psychotherapy.

Interestingly enough, the treatment for this syndrome is still supportive psychotherapy and mild tranquilizers, even if the symptoms are found to be due to brain injury. The patient with difficulty concentrating and fatigability, needs encouragement to engage in his former activities and work, and he needs reassurance that the symptoms will subside in time.

TUBERCULOSIS

Although the incidence of TB is declining in the United States, it is still prevalent in underpriviledged areas and among alcoholics.

When I was working the emergency room in psychiatry one evening, an alcoholic was sent to see me, not because he had a problem with his alcoholism, but because he had vague pain in the upper right side of his chest. (Why this should be cause for him to be told to see the psychiatrist remains a mystery.) This patient said he had a pain in the upper right side of his chest which hurt when he breathed in deeply. I asked if he had lost weight recently, and indeed he had lost 15 pounds in the last two months. I asked if he had night sweats, where he would almost drench the bed, and he replied that he often had to get up during the night to change his pajamas due to their wetness from sweating. He also said he had been more tired lately, and had a cough which he said he always had and which he attributed to excessive smoking. I ordered a chest x-ray. The patient had TB.

The preceding note about TB is included in this chapter on anxiety because of the association of night sweating with both entities. Chronically anxious patients often awake in a cold sweat in the middle of the night. Their anxiety often makes them persistently fatigued during the day. The triad of night sweating, chronic fatigue, and recent weight loss should alert you to send the patient for a check-up before treating him for anxiety.

PHEOCHROMOCYTOMA

A pheochromocytoma is a type of tumor which elaborates epinephrine and norepinephrine—the chemicals which participate in the making of a sympathetic reaction and an anxiety reaction that were discussed early in this chapter. It is an *extremely* rare tumor, but symptomatically presents itself as anxiety, excessive sweating, and headaches—a not uncommon psychological triad. Further manifestations are again those described for anxiety states: subjective nervousness, tremors, rapid heartbeat, nausea, weakness, and occasional chest or abdominal pain.

In general, someone complaining of persistent headaches along with symptoms of anxiety should be referred to an M.D.

You can never be 100% certain (always think tumor)! I once had a patient who complained of extremely short bouts of anxiety, occurring almost daily, lasting five minutes or so. She could never pinpoint exactly what set these off, but while they lasted she was terribly distressed and somewhat confused. She had been from doctor to doctor for over a year, and every one of them had told her to see a psychiatrist. Finally, she remembered to tell one astute M.D. that she smelled something funny before each attack and that she had noticed that the vision in her right eye wasn't as good as it used to be. It turned out she had a brain tumor whose first manifestation was anxiety attacks.

There are *many other* medical and/or neurological diseases which have anxiety symptoms included in the picture. Generally speaking therefore, it is a good idea for all patients to have a general medical checkup early in the course of their psychotherapy.

CHAPTER II

Psychophysiologic Disorders

The term psychosomatic is used commonly, and is thought by the general public to be a disorder that is "all in your head." The term is often used incorrectly to describe almost delusional ideas or bodily complaints for which no medical basis can be found. The term psychophysiological better describes the complex interaction of psychological and physiological factors which make up these disorders. Psychophysiologic disorders are defined in the "Diagnostic and Statistical Manual of the American Psychiatric Association" as *physical* disorders of *presumably* psychogenic origin. We have already come across a disorder which is considered to be psychophysiological, namely the hyperventilation syndrome. There, as in the case of the disorders discussed in this chapter, psychological factors play a role in producing a state of altered physiology in the body. In other words, psychophysiological disorders are "real" in the sense that they have actual physical SIGNS of disease (such as the real ulcer hole in the stomach lining) and actual physical *SYMPTOMS* (such as tension headache or extreme difficulty in breathing as in asthma) which are produced by altered physiology in the body. These disorders are recognized as having heavy psychological components but it has *NEVER* been demonstrated that psychological factors *ALONE* can cause any of them. Psychological stress is known to be able to set off (as in asthma) or considerably aggravate the underlying physical or physiological condition which predisposes the individual to the disorder in question. Let me repeat, however, that psychological factors *alone* are not solely responsible for psychophysiologic diseases nor can these conditions be treated by psychological means alone. Psychotherapy can help reduce the frequency of asthmatic attacks or attacks of ulcerative colitis, but the therapist, and indeed the patient, should always remain in communication with the patient's medical doctor. In order to better understand psychophysiologic diseases, it is helpful to know that there is another network of nerves in the body known as the parasympathetic nervous system.* The neurotransmitter for this whole system is acetylcholine, hence the term cholinergic system (choline = abbreviation for acetylcholine; ergic = moved by). The functions of the cholinergic system involve: slowing the heart rate; decreasing the diameter of the bronchi (breathing tubes); regulating the amount of stomach acid; keeping the food moving through the intestines (by consecutively constricting and relaxing section after section of the intestines (peristalsis); maintaining an erection; and opening urinary and anal sphincters to allow urination and defecation. There are many other functions but they do not concern us here.

It is interesting that one very large and long nerve which originates in the brain controls many of the functions we have just mentioned. This is the vagus nerve and its branches which supply the heart, stomach, and all of the intestines up until the last half of the "large intestine" (colon). Other parasympathetic nerves which originate in the spinal cord control erection (to a certain extent) and bladder and bowel elimination. This is valuable knowledge since many drugs, especially major tranquilizers (see Chapter 8)

---

*The parasympathetic nervous system, like the sympathetic system, is really a part of the body's whole nervous system, but it too can be affected as a whole (by various drugs or psychological reactions).

and certain antidepressants of the tricyclic type (see Chapter 9) are *anti*cholinergic. That is, they interfere with the functioning of the cholinergic system and cause such things as rapid heart rate, constipation, inability to get an erection, and difficulty in starting urination to name a few. These anticholinergic side effects of the tranquilizers and antidepressants will be taken up again with their respective drugs. However, it is also important for you to know about the parasympathetic (cholinergic) system for another reason and that is that *emotions* and thoughts can affect the system, particularly the vagus nerve, and can contribute to the development of ulcers and ulcerative colitis, "irritable colon" syndrome, and asthma, which are generally considered the major psychophysiologic disorders.

In general, the parasympathetic and sympathetic nervous systems are antagonistic in the actions they produce. Whereas pulses along the parasympathetic fibers to the heart for example, can cause it to slow down, a sympathetic pulsing can cause increased heart rate. This principle can be used pharmacologically in very elegant ways to control some of the symptoms of the diseases which are about to be discussed.

ASTHMA

Asthma is a very complex psychophysiologic disorder. It is generally agreed that psychological stress can trigger off an asthmatic attack, but the patient has many physiologic predispositions which are highly contributory. Often the asthmatic patient is predisposed to allergies of many kinds and contact with any substance to which he is allergic can also trigger an attack in the absence of psychological stress. An asthmatic attack is an extremely anxiety-producing experience in and of itself because the patient feels like he cannot breathe, that he is suffocating and is going to die. What actually happens is that there is severe constriction of the bronchi. The drug used to treat an acute attack is, a *sympathetic* nervous system stimulant, epinephrine—which you may remember is secreted by the adrenal glands in times of stress and causes a sympathetic reaction, one component of which is opening of the bronchi. Drugs used to prevent asthmatic attacks often contain sympathetic stimulants for the same reason and these can make an asthmatic patient chronically irritable, nervous, anxious, and insomniac. It is therefore terribly important that the asthmatic patient be asked what, if any, medications he is taking for asthma, before assuming he has excessive anxiety. Unfortunately, many asthmatic patients are quite chronically anxious anyway. It is best that the asthmatic's doctor prescribe minor tranquilizers like chlordiazepoxide (Librium) or diazepam (Valium) because major ones (phenothiazines, See Chapter 8) tend to cause constriction of the bronchi and predispose the taker to more asthmatic attacks.

As you can see, treating asthmatics is very tricky and should really be jointly handled by a psychiatrist and an internist. However when working with an asthmatic patient you should be alert to the anxiety-causing properties of antiasthmatic medicines and the asthma-attack predisposing potential of major tranquilizers and antidepressants. It is also necessary to realize and also inform the patient that psychotherapy itself can temporarily cause stress which may further aggravate asthmatic attacks.

ULCERS

An ulcer is an erosion of part of the lining of the stomach or the duodenum (part of the intestine just after the stomach). An ulcer is really quite small, often less than one-half inch in diameter. One of its characteristic symptoms is that eating most foods (except spices and onions, etc.), especially milk-derived foods, relieves the chronic pain which is usually located on the right side or midline, just below the rib cage. Ulcers are also a very complex psychophysiologic disorder. It is known that ulcer patients have a higher amount of acid in their stomachs than the rest of the population. All the mechanisms which come together to cause an ulcer are not yet fully understood, but one highly contributory factor appears to be overactivity of the vagus nerve's branches to the stomach. (If you remember, the vagus nerve originates in the brain and by extremely complex mechanisms is influenced by thought and emotion.) The surgeon often cuts the vagus nerve's branches to the stomach if an operation is necessary for an ulcer. In this case, the anticholinergic properties of major tranquilizers and antidepressants are in the patient's favor but the gastric (stomach) irritation produced by those drugs themselves are not. Again they are probably better off with minor tranquilizers, if tranquilizers are necessary.

Ulcers can bleed if the erosion hits a blood vessel. If the bleeding is slow but significant *over time* the patient may begin to complain of weakness, fatigue, depression or anxiety *which are also signs of anemia*. Be alert to this if your patient *has* an ulcer or has *ever* had one, since they are prone to recurrence even though they heal. A patient with a history of an ulcer who keeps his appointment with you having awakened with severe anxiety, rapid heart rate, cold sweating, weakness and/or nausea and who, *if you remember to ask*, admits to having had a black tarry diarrhea-like stool that morning should be taken to a hospital since he is showing signs of acute blood loss. (In this case the sympathetic reaction was set off by severe blood loss.) Many neurotic ulcer patients get into psychological panics and severe anxiety reactions which have the same symptoms as just described for acute blood loss. In this situation, check with the patient about having a black unformed bowel movement or vomiting blood. If neither have occurred it is unlikely that the patient is suffering severe blood loss. The slow blood loss causing anemia is a little trickier since it might not be noticed in the stool, and all that remains is fatigue, depression, and other "psychological" symptoms. It is always wise to have the patient, with an ulcer history, who complains of fatigue and depression, check with his internist before continuing or initiating either psychotherapy or antidepressants.

ULCERATIVE COLITIS

Ulcerative colitis is a condition of small ulcerations and severe inflammation of the colon (large intestine). It is characterized by intermittent bouts, lasting days to months, of constant diarrhea which is often bloody. Psychological and physiological components both play major roles in this disorder. It can be debilitating and can lead to death by several mechanisms. The patient with this disease currently, or even with a history of it, who wants psychotherapy *must* be treated by a psychiatrist and an internist simultaneously and no nonmedical psychotherapist should undertake treatment for such a patient.* Psychotherapy itself is, of necessity, often very stressful to the patient. This could set off a fulminating attack of quiescent ulcerative colitis which could end in severe physical debilitation of the patient, if not bring him close to death.

IMPOTENCE

Never assume that impotence is psychologically caused until the man has been checked out thoroughly by a doctor. There are some screening medical questions you can ask which may save a lot of time. Of course a good psychosexual history is in order.

The maintenance of an erection is a psychophysiologic function involving the parasympathetic (cholinergic) nervous system. The ability to ejaculate is a psychophysiologic function involving the sympathetic nervous system. Strictly speaking the inability to achieve or maintain an erection is known as impotence, and the inability to ejaculate is known as ejaculatory incompetence. If a patient is complaining of either of these problems, the *first thing* to ask him is about his *intake* of *alcohol* and/or drugs or medicines. The most common cause of sudden impotence in a previously potent man is over-indulgence in alcohol. Alcohol, by many mechanisms, can prevent erection, and a cycle of impotence is begun in the following way. The man has too much to drink one night, wants to have intercourse and finds that he can't get an erection. This is extremely upsetting to him especially if it is the first time it ever happened. He vows to try to have intercourse the next night, so beforehand to calm himself down he has a few shots, maybe a few too many and lo and behold "it" won't "work" again. After that, he is so worried that "it" won't "work", that he can't (sometimes) get an erection even without the alcohol, and comes to a therapist in a panic. So it is always advisable to ask such a patient how much liquor he usually drinks before attempt-

---

*This really has to do with the sociology of medicine in the sense that it is usually easier for an M.D. to keep in constant communication with another M.D. than it is for a lay therapist to do so. If, however, you have very good continuous communication between you and the patient's internist, it is certainly okay to initiate psychotherapy.

ing intercourse and especially how much he drank the night that his erective competence first failed. Theoretically, many drugs could cause impotence if they have anticholinergic properties. Since phenothiazines are both anticholinergic and antisympathetic they could cause both impotence and ejaculatory incompetence. I have, however, more often heard of difficulty in ejaculation than difficulty with erection. The anticholinergic properties seem to be taken out on the urinary sphincter since difficulty in starting urination is another common complaint with phenothiazines and tricyclic antidepressants.

Impotence can also result from a host of medical and neurological diseases such as diabetes, alcoholic neuropathy, advanced syphilis, multiple sclerosis, and many others. Therefore, it is a good idea to have the patient checked out medically before proceeding with psychotherapy.

Heroin is a notorious cause for either impotence or delayed or completely inhibited ejaculation. Another occurrence reported with certain phenothiazines is that a man has an orgasm but no semen is emitted—this can really be cause for panic in a person already in need of major tranquilizers. What may happen is that occasionally there may occur a retrograde ejaculation back into the man's bladder rather than out through his penis. That is, for as yet unexplained reasons, the usual direction of the seminal emission is reversed, and the semen is propelled into the bladder rather than out. The gratification of orgasm remains however with the exception of the enjoyment derived from the actual sensation of the semen leaving the penis. It so happens that this phenomenon has been more often reported with thioridazine and mesoridazine although it is known to occur with all phenothiazines. Very often there are compelling reasons, however, to use these particular phenothiazines. If this happens to one of your patients, and you can explain that it is a side effect of the drug, and, moreover, remind him that he is still having an orgasm, he may well be willing to live with it. It is also of great importance to reassure him that there is nothing wrong with *him*.

There are as many psychological causes for impotence as there are men who have the difficulty. It is only necessary to realize that there may be drug or alcohol-related causes or medical diseases which need to be ruled out before the sometimes difficult psycho-therapeutic job of relieving the impotence is undertaken.

PREMENSTRUAL TENSION SYNDROME

Mild depression, irritability, headache, fluid retention (water bloating), breast and/or abdominal tenderness, a few days to a week before menstruation have a normal physiologic basis. Menstrual cramps, not severe enough to require narcotics, also have a physiologic basis. The mild depression and cramps, etc. have for too long been considered as neurotic symptoms having as their "unconscious roots" the rejection of femininity by the woman who experiences them. This is nonsense. It is medically and psychologically wrong to consider these symptoms as neurotic—*within reasonable limits.* There *are*, however, women, who for a variety of either *medical or unconscious* reasons, experience unusually severe menstrual cramps and premenstrual symptoms. It is wise to have the woman check with her gynecologist, especially if menstrual cramping is severe enough to incapacitate her from work, etc. Women in our society have been allowed to use this as an excuse for time off, even though it is not necessary. What is meant here is *incapacitating* cramps which prevent the woman from doing whatever she *wanted* to do. Women, in our society, are also allowed to react, or overreact to pain, so it is difficult to get a good idea of how much of a psycho-logical component there is to the premenstrual tension syndrome or menstrual cramps, versus how much of anything of true gynecologic origin. If premenstrual "tension" or other symptoms appear to be playing a disproportionate part in the woman's sociosexual relations, a gynecological examination is definitely in order.

FRIGIDITY

Frigidity is a very complex psychophysiologic disorder. Strictly speaking there can be failure of any arousal at all, which would manifest itself physically as lack of engorgement of the labia and lack of lubrication of the vagina. There can also be arousal with failure to have orgasm, which by itself is a complex psychophysiologic function. If I may interpret some of the deluge of literature on this subject, it seems that the most common cause for either failure of arousal or failure of orgasm is inadequate or improper stimulation. That is, that the partners of so-called frigid women may not know how or particularly where or when to sexually stimulate these women. Therefore, in dealing with a so-called frigid woman, a particularly detailed psychosexual history is in order.

It is known that some of the physiologic functions involved in arousal and orgasm are under the control of the sympathetic and parasympathetic nerves of the lower spinal cord. So that any diseases previously listed for men, which affect the lower spinal cord, could affect orgastic capacity in women. These nerves also have endings which supply the uterus. *Small* uterine contractions are therefore a natural part of orgasm. *They, in no way, endanger a normal pregnancy at any stage.*

Although definitive studies showing the labial and vaginal responses to drugs are lacking, I have heard of both major tranquilizers and antidepressants causing a decrease in vaginal lubrication during sexual stimulation. Certainly CNS depressants could depress libido and cause frigidity on that psychophysiologic basis. In general, the same warning is given here as was given for men. Never assume a woman is frigid on psychological grounds until she has been checked by her gynecologist and probably *also* her internist. One further note. Never assume a woman is frigid until the pattern of stimulation by her partner is thoroughly detailed.

CHAPTER III

Depression

Feelings of depression are probably the most commonly encountered complaints in the outpaitient practice of psychotherapy. It is necessary at the outset, therefore, to distinguish between a clinically *significant* depression which today *can* and *must* be treated with drugs, and a minor feeling of depression which can safely be treated with psychotherapy alone.

Clinically significant depressions are associated with *biological* as well as *psychological* manifestations. It has been shown that depression with biological signs are associated with much higher suicide rates than those which do not have biological signs. Furthermore, patients with *recurrent* depressive episodes (who never experience hypomania), who are called *unipolar* depressives, and patients with recurrent attacks of depression which are interlaced with recurrent attacks of excessively good mood and overactivity (hypomania or mania), who are called *bipolar* or manic-depressive patients, have a 10 to 20 times higher suicide rate than the general population. Both these groups have biological signs.

What are biological signs?: sleep disorders, appetite disorders, and psychomotor symptoms. Each of these will be described below. The important thing to realize is that depressions *with* biological signs *are* quite serious, and that they are more likely to respond to drug therapy, which makes it doubly imperative that these patients be referred to a psychiatrist (in preference to general practitioner) for appropriate medication.

DISORDERS OF SLEEP

Early morning awakening

The patient, although going to bed at his usual time, wakes up consistantly much earlier (2-4 hours earlier) than his usual awakening time and *cannot* get back to sleep.

Intermittent wakefulness

The patient can't stay asleep long, sleeps a few hours, is awake for an hour or two, falls back to sleep and wakes again. It is important to realize that the total time spent asleep may not be shortened if the patient spends long enough in bed, but his sleep is disrupted.

Difficulty falling asleep

This can be a sign of anxiety as well as depression and is usually combined with other sleep disturbance in severe depression. Sometimes, in severe depression, all three difficulties are present and the patient has nearly complete insomnia.

Hypersomnia

The patient sleeps excessively (9-12 hours) during the night, and often during the day, claiming this to be his only respite from depressed mood. It is important to realize that this type of sleep disorder, along with other biological, psychological and historical signs, can be a *biological* sign of depression and not merely an "escapist mechanism."

APPETITE DISORDERS

The incidence of depression increases with increasing age in males and females. Generally, middle-aged patients who are experiencing their first major depression, and unipolar recurrent depressives, have *loss* of appetite (anorexia) and subsequent weight loss. However, some bipolar patients, and often chronically obese patients, respond to depression with overeating and weight gain. If the depression has been going on for one month or more, a significant (10 lb. or more) weight loss or weight gain will usually have occurred.

PSYCHOMOTOR SYMPTOMS

Psychomotor retardation

The patient will have a monotonous facial expression; he may remain in one position for a prolonged period of time (15 minutes or more); he does not use his hands in talking, and they may remain in his lap or on the arms of the chair; his sentences may be halting, with much time elapsing between them or even between words of a sentence. The clinician gets the impression of a general slowness to the patient's thought processes, speech, and movements.

Psychomotor agitation

More easily observable than retardation, psychomotor agitation involves inability to sit still, pacing, wringing of hands, frequent changes (or contortions) of facial expressions and body positions, and excessive, rapid talking. The clinician here gets the impression of an extreme restlessness, and hyperactivity of the patient's body movements, thought processes, and speech.

Anergia

This differs somewhat from psychomotor retardation, in that the person shows severe lack of energy. The slightest usual act like brushing hair may be felt to be too much to accomplish for the patient with this symptom. The patient with retardation, however, will brush her hair but *very* slowly. Usually this symptom is associated with hypersomnia, and together they are becoming recognized as often characteristic of the manic-depressive (bipolar) type of depression.

OTHER PSYCHOBIOLOGICAL SIGNS

Loss of libido

This means usually, loss of sexual interest, but it may be accompanied by impotence or frigidity as well. In a broader sense it refers to loss of interest in most things in the world outside the self. A loss of emotional investment in people, activities, etc.

Anhedonia

This is a bit different from loss of libido although it does overlap with it. It is the inability to experience pleasure from any source, as well as the loss of the pleasure seeking drive. People with this symptom literally can't think of anything that would give them pleasure, nor do they experience pleasure from any person or activity.

These, then, are the biological signs associated with *clinically significant* depressions: sleep disorder—too little or too much sleep; appetite disorder—more frequently loss of appetite but bipolars and chronically obese may have increased appetite; psychomotor symptoms—either retardation or agitation or hyperactivity and loss of drive. It is *not* necessary for all of these to be present to make the diagnosis. If it is cause for more than 3 hours loss of sleep per night, a sleep disorder *alone, combined with psychological symptoms* of depression, is sufficient evidence of significant, drug-treatable depression. (Technically speaking there occasionally occurs a severely depressed person without a clinically apparent sleep disorder, but he will show other signs of severe depression such as marked psychomotor retardation. It has been shown, however, that these patients do have a sleep disorder manifest on their sleeping EEG (electroencephalograph) records.)

The psychological signs of depression are much more familiar. The patient may complain of being unable to enjoy anything; loss of sexual desire and/or capacity for orgasm, sadness, indecisiveness, irritability, and impaired memory, especially for recent events. Very frequently they have feelings of total personal inadequacy, combined with a hopelessness and a helplessness in which they perceive themselves as beyond help from anyone including the therapist or medications. Suicidal thoughts are very frequent, so frequent in fact, that if patients who *have biological signs* of depression deny these thoughts they should be suspected of harboring them with the intention of acting on them, and hence, considered an even greater suicide risk.

One further note about biological signs. Sleep disorders can be masked if the patient regularly uses alcohol, sleeping-pills or narcotics. Even the psychological extent of the depression can be masked by the temporary euphoric effect of alcohol or narcotics. The worst thing about alcohol, sleeping-pills, and narcotics in depression, is that they increase the depression, although the patient may continue to take them for the *temporary* relief they afford. *Therefore, be alert especially to the patient who has increased his use of these drugs, while continuing to complain of psychological symptoms of depression,* even if he has no evident sleep or appetite disorder.

BRIEF CLASSIFICATION OF DEPRESSIONS

I once had a patient transferred to me from another therapist who had seen her intensively for a year, for depression, but had never considered to refer her for a course of antidepressants. When I saw the patient she was tearful most of the session, complained of severe anergia and said she slept nine or ten hours per night plus whatever other times she could. She said that sleeping was all she ever wanted to do, maybe sleep forever. She said her marriage was fine but she felt she was becoming a burden to her husband because of her depression. She doubted if he could stand much more of it even though he had been so tolerant up to that point. (I might add here that this is a very frequent complaint by depressed people. That is, that they are burdening their loved ones. Such thoughts present a good reason for suicide and as such constitute a serious symptom—whether or not they are true.) I asked her if she had ever had "high" periods, excessively high, where she would be very busy with many projects, happy-go-lucky, spend too much money in sprees, or have increased sexual drive. She answered that she had been like she was now (depressed) for the last two years and had always been depressed her whole life. I started her on antidepressants and about three weeks later, again questioned her about possible high periods. This time she indeed remembered that she had had a sexual affair on the spur of the moment (very unusual for her) just before she met her husband. She added that she was so bubbly that she was the only one who could "draw her husband out" (he was the quiet shy type). She recalled going on a spending spree during that period and said that she would sing to herself at work, write poetry and paint after work. She said that this lasted for about six months, whereupon, just before getting married she became depressed, and had remained depressed since. Notice that she was so depressed in the first interview that it colored her whole view of her own history, so that she did not recall the high period at that time. This patient was suffering from manic-depressive *ILLNESS, NOT NECESSARILY PSYCHOSIS.* The concept of manic-depressive *illness* has been developed in United States Psychiatry so as to include patients who never become psychotic, but suffer from periodic bouts of moderate to severe hypomanic or manic episodes and moderate to severe depressive episodes, *accompanied* by *biological signs.* Those patients with psychotic symptoms during the mood swings (such as hallucinations, delusions or inability to meet ordinary demands of life) are said to have the manic-depressive *psychosis.* Those patients with mild mood swings are called cyclothymic personalities. Increasingly the term bipolar is being used to describe this illness *or* psychosis. The biological signs of manic or hypomanic episodes are accelerated speech and motor activity, irritability, and loss of sleep. These are accompanied by excessive elation, talkativeness and flight of ideas (patient goes from one subject to the next very rapidly), increased sexual drive, increased interest in many activities simultaneously, in general a complete reversal of what occurs in depression. In acute delirious, psychotic mania the patient may become incoherent, delusional, and possibly hallucinate.

The biological signs of the depression of manic-depressive illness are severe psychomotor retardation (although sometimes psychomotor agitation is present) sleep loss or sleep excess, severe anergia and anhedonia. These are accompanied by severely depressed mood, occassionally including delusions or hallucinations.

Indeed, it can often be very difficult, especially in delirious mania, to differentiate between "loosening of associations" such as occurs in schizophrenia and extreme flight of ideas of the mania. Luckily, most of these patients will not be likely to come to an outpatient setting, or be seen by a non-M.D. psychotherapist first. Often actual differentiation can only be made after several episodes and an assessment of the quality of the interim periods.

The term *unipolar* describes patients without a clear-cut history of hypomanic or manic behavior, but who suffer from periodic bouts of depression with biological signs. In general postpartum depression (psychosis), psychotic depressive reactions, and involutional melancholia are the standard diagnostic labels which are here being subsumed under the term unipolar. In addition patients who experience their first major depression in middle age or later with *no* anecdent history of hypomania or mania (no matter how far in the past) are generally similar to the unipolar group in their response to drug therapy.

In any event, it is obvious how important a good history is when speaking to a depressed patient, and as is the case with the patient described, how difficult it may be to get a good history when the patient is severely depressed.

Biopolar patients *tend* to have hypersomnia and severe anergia albeit sometimes with increased appetite when they are depressed. Unipolar and "first-depressions of middle age" or psychotic depressive reactions tend to have insomnia, anorexia, and variable psychomotor symptoms. In either event, the depression has biological signs and this should be the signal to have the patient seen by a psychiatrist who can prescribe the appropriate medication. Generally, bipolar patients are treated with either tricyclic antidepressants or MAO inhibitors (see Chapter 9) and lithium salts to lessen manic attacks and prevent depression once the anti-depressants have worked.

There is a growing body of evidence also that lithium may possibly work by itself as an antidepressant in manic-depressive depression. Unipolar patients tend to respond very well to tri-cyclics for their depression in combination with major or minor tranquilizers for any agitation present.

When depression is related specifically to a precipitating cause and is associated with delusions, hallucinations or other psychotic symptoms, the patient is said to be psychotically depressed (technically denoted as a psychotic depressive reaction). Depression also occurs in schizophrenic syndromes and it may be difficult to distinguish at first between a psychotically depressed person and a depressed schizophrenic. The differentiation is made on the basis of age, history, and several other factors. Psychotic depressive reaction is often associated with somatic delusions (delusions concerning the body). That is, the patient believes there is something physically wrong with him, that he has cancer, that he is going to die, or that some organ or system in his body is rotting. Sometimes these delusions approximate the symptomatic description of a real physical illness. It is important, therefore, to have such a patient checked by a psychiatrist who might more easily distinguish between complaints which could have an anatomic basis, and those that most likely do not.

One further note on this subject. Sadness, psychomotor retar-dation, weight loss, insomnia, mild memory impairment, anergia or chronic fatigue, irritability, and vague or specific somatic com-plaints can all be signs of an as yet undiscovered physical illness. Medical consultation is imperative in patients with these psycho-biological signs and symptoms. The final pages of this chapter present possible alternatives to a diagnosis of depression.

HYPOTHYROIDISM

Every once in a while I am reminded of the importance of *looking* at a patient. A patient came to me complaining of depression and said she had gained forty pounds in the last four months. Her sleep pattern was normal and she had no psycho-motor symptoms. She was not a binge eater, and had never previously been fat. She was a smoker, and had a somewhat deep voice for a woman, which she thought had always been that way. Somewhere out of my previous medical training came the thought of hypothyroidism (probably based on nothing more than the weight gain). *Then*, I took a look at her. She had no hair on the outer third of her eyebrows and no hair on her legs, and she didn't shave or tweeze either one. The characteristic changes of hypothyroidism were right there: obesity, loss of leg hair and the peculiarly characteristic loss of eyebrow hair on the outer third of both eyebrows, and very characteristically a deep voice.

Hypothyroidism is *under*activity of the thyroid gland. These patients complain of depression, loss of energy, chronic fatigue or weakness just like depressed patients. Also, females may have only a few or no menstrual periods, a symptom consonant with either hypothyroidism or depression. Most people have usually gained a considerable amount of weight, inexplicably, if the disease has been going on for a few months. In addition to the hair losses, deep voice, and obesity, they have a tendency to feel cold or be sensitive to cold weather. A good look at your patient and a careful listening to his/her voice in addition to a history of weight gain and depression should alert you to the possibility of hypothyroidism along with the possibility of a clinically significant depression.

ADDISON'S DISEASE

Addison's Disease is a relatively rare disease of the adrenal glands, and is mentioned very briefly because its onset is characterized by the same psychological and biological signs as depression. The one outstanding characteristic to be aware of is a deep tanning of the skin which occurs with or without exposure to the sun. If you happen to notice a particularly deep tan on a patient who complains of depression, fatigability, anorexia, etc. it wouldn't hurt to check it out with an internist.

DEPRESSION SECONDARY TO VARIOUS DRUGS

As mentioned, alcohol, sleeping-pills, and narcotics are ultimately depressing drugs even if they produce temporary

euphoria. In addition, persons addicted to their use very often have chronic depressions for which they use those drugs. Antidepressants can be used even in the face of alcohol, sleeping-pills or narcotic abuse, but dosage and patient reliability are problems not easily solved.

Not so infrequent causes for depression are drugs used in the treatment of high blood pressure, and this must be kept in mind when a patient complains of depression. The worst offender in this category is Reserpine or drugs derived from Reserpine or containing Reserpine, commonly known as Serpasil, Raudixin, Renese, Regroton, Hydromox, Diupres, etc. These and another antihypertensive, alpha-methyldopa (Aldomet), can cause severe psychological depression in about 15% of those persons treated with them, and who may or may not exhibit biological signs. *The importance of asking the patient what drugs or medications he is taking*, before even thinking about psychological causes for his distress, *cannot be overemphasized.* Drugs given as tranquilizers, such as meprobamate (Miltown, Equanil), diazepam (Valium), chlordiazepoxide (Librium), or even phenothiazines (Thorazine, Stelazine, Trilafon, etc.) can cause or worsen depressed mood. Amphetamines, (speed) commonly thought to be "ups" or stimulants, are responsible for depression also. It has been shown experimentally that when volunteers were given large doses, they became depressed (before becoming psychotic, I might add). Furthermore, when amphetamine "highs" wear off, the person commonly experiences a "let-down" which can be a severe depression depending on how high a dose he was taking before he stopped. In street language, the tremendous depression following discontinuance of chronic ingestion of amphetamines is known as "crashing." This type of depression can be quite severe and presents a moderate suicide risk.

In summary then, depressed mood can occur in a wide variety of psychological and medical situations. Biological signs such as sleep and appetite disorders and psychomotor symptoms occur almost always in clinically significant depressions, and indicate a more serious depression than psychological depression without those signs. The suicide rate among depressives with biological signs is vastly higher than for the general population. Depressions with biological signs require drug therapy even if the signs have only been present for two weeks. (A patient who loses some sleep on one or two nights, however, is not ordinarily an immediate candidate for antidepressants. Nor, is the person who has had life-long feelings of depression without accompanying biological signs.)

Antidepressant drug therapy *works* in the range of 60-70% of the time, with some estimates even higher, hence it is truly tragic to treat a psychobiologically depressed person solely with psycho-therapy, when a great deal of his misery could be alleviated in two or three weeks. Such therapy might even prevent a suicide.

CHAPTER IV

Does Your Patient Have "Organic" Brain Disorder

The concept of organic brain disorder includes several constellations of symptoms which doctors have come to recognize are associated with *damage to or loss of actual nerve cells* in the brain or disturbance in their transmission of impulses. When the damage, loss or dysfunction is diffuse throughout the brain, certain characteristic symptoms appear which can be recognized as associated with this organic damage. (Organic refers to the *organ* involved, specifically, the brain.) These characteristic symptoms occur together often enough to be called a syndrome (constellation of symptoms). They occur together regardless of the cause of the damage to the nerve cells (neurons), if the damage is *diffuse*. If the damage is localized, as in psychomotor seizures, it is given the name of the area involved (psychomotor seizures = temporal lobe epilepsy = "uncinate fits". Uncinate refers to the uncus which is a smaller area within the temporal lobe of the brain.)

Regardless of the cause of known or even unknown damage to the brain, the symptoms are called an organic brain syndrome (OBS for short). An OBS may occur with or without psychosis. If the OBS *itself* prevents the patient from meeting the ordinary demands of life or from knowing reality it is considered an OBS with psychosis. *Whenever you find the symptoms of organic brain disease*, it should cause you to *immediately refer the patient to an M.D.*, preferably a *psychiatrist* or *neurologist*.

Diagnosing organic brain disease is easy in some cases but can be confusing in others. For example, acute schizophrenics are often confused, do not know the date, are disoriented and in general may present many "organic" features. It may not be possible to tell if this is permanent or temporary until the psychotic symptoms are under control. In other cases, where clear metabolic or circulatory disturbances are known to be present or have occurred, or head injury or drug ingestion has clearly preceded the presence of "organic" symptoms, the diagnosis is easier. Especially with regard to organic brain disorders, it is imperative that the patient be questioned about drug and alcohol ingestion.

The cardinal signs of organic brain syndrome due to *diffuse* impairment of neurons are: impairment of memory, orientation, intellect, judgment, and lability of affect. (Lability of affect is a state where the person very quickly changes from one affect to another; for example, from fear of the examiner to love of the examiner or from tears to laughter, etc.)

IMPAIRMENT OF MEMORY

The earliest signs of memory impairment may be simply tossed off as absent-mindedness. The person is beginning to forget the most recent events of his life or most recent things he was saying. Yet, there is often remarkable preservation for past memories in this early phase. The difficulty really seems at first limited to the neurons responsible for learning and retaining the newest information. Later on, difficulty in remembering past events becomes greater, until ultimately little of the past or present is retained.

Depressives of whatever classification and some neurotics, as well as persons with major psychoses, will complain of difficulty with recent memory. Close questioning, however, will almost always, reveal this to be due to difficulties they have been having with concentration; a problem which, however, can also be a sign of organic impairment. Severely depressed persons or others with major psychoses may not even be concentrating enough on the present to be forming their "recent-memory traces" because they are preoccupied with their psychological difficulties. Persons in older age groups may blame their memory difficulties on getting old, when they are really due to depression or other "functional" problems. It is important therefore, not to assume someone is "organic" based on age alone, and to defer the diagnosis of organicity until the depression or other symptoms have been controlled. There are several ways of testing these memory functions. Much testing can be accomplished with the taking of the history of the present illness. In other words, as the patient describes his difficulties take note of whether he keeps saying "I can't remember" with respect to recent events or past events. The striking thing is that all of us have difficulty in remembering the past, but patients with true OBS have difficulty remembering the present or most recent past. There are specific ways to test this function of memory; these are listed under "formal mental status" in Chapter 6.

IMPAIRMENT OF ORIENTATION

The earliest signs of orientation impairment are difficulties in remembering time sequences of events, despite the fact that the patient can remember the events themselves. If there is progression of disorientation, the patient will begin to forget the events themselves, or more particularly, where and when the events took place. In general, orientation is divided into three sub-categories—time, place, and person. Disorientation to time is an earlier finding, i.e., a more acute finding, than is disorientation to place or person. What is meant by time disorientation is not only the actual time of day, but *what* day, month, season, year, it is. Later on, with further impairment, difficulty in knowing where he is or who the examiner is may occur, and ultimately, after almost all functions of memory and orientation have failed, the patient will be unable to tell you who he himself is. There are many

degrees of knowing where one is. In general this question of place-
ment refers to where the patient is at the moment the question is
asked. Obviously not just "in a room" or a vague or nonspecific
answer, but an answer indicating the title of the place like
hospital, doctor's office, emergency room, clinic, etc. is desired.

With respect to orientation to person, this really means does the
patient recognize persons previously known to him by name or
correct relationship, and persons unknown to him by title or
function. Remember, only after all functions of orientation and
memory have failed, will a person be unable to tell you who he
himself is. (Hysterics will feign or really be unable to remember
who they are, but there will be no consistent pattern of total
memory loss and orientation loss to go along with this type of
orientation failure.) The cardinal questions to be answered by the
patient either directly or in your mind are: does the patient know
what day, month, and year this is, *where* he is, who *you* are, not
your name necessarily, but your functional title (e.g., examiner,
nurse, worker, doctor, etc.) and lastly, who he is. More subtly,
does the patient know the sequence of events from yesterday to
today which led to his coming to see you (if this is the first interview) or what occurred during yesterday. Questions to test
orientation are part of the formal mental status as outlined in
Chapter 6.

IMPAIRMENT OF JUDGMENT

Judgement impairment can be subtle or can be the purpose for
which the patient has found himself in your office. This problem is
difficult to describe since judgment itself is often a value-laden
subjective thing anyway. In general judgment can be assessed by
evaluating whether or not the person violated his own usual code
of behavior or values, or whether he did or said something which
is not customary for his socioeconomic class. That is pretty broad,
and must therefore be tempered by other factors, such as whether
the person was deliberately rebelling against these value systems,
or whether indeed he was, for example, so euphoric that he bought
a $20,000 dollar car when he makes $15,000 dollars per year.
Here, however, we are really considering *gross* judgmental im-

pairment such as not being able to assess that 30 degrees Fahrenheit is sufficiently cold out to warrant more than shirt sleeves. General states of dress or undress are usually functions of judgment. This is often impaired in schizophrenia and therefore by itself should not be considered significant of an OBS. The old, "What would you do if you found a stamped unopened letter in the street?" is really unfair for judgment, but is a good index of sociopathy. Generally, your assessment of the patient's judgment will have to come from outside sources if his impairment is more subtle than what is described here. It usually involves slow but noticeable inattention to obvious considerations in decision making and may lead to persons beginning to see the patient as unreliable.

IMPAIRMENT OF INTELLECT

Intellect impairment is more easily directly testable by proverbs, numbers, similarities, etc. than described. Essentially, however, a person's vocabulary and interests may decline. He may not be able to intellectually deal with more than one idea simultaneously, which is a cardinal sign of higher intellect regardless of his level of intelligence as long as it is average. The signs of intellectual impairment may be reported by outside sources, or become subtly evident during discussion with the patient. Impairment of intellect also depends to a great extent upon the environmental demands placed upon the patient. I heard of a case of a scientist who could no longer do higher-order calculus. This was the first sign of his intellectual impairment. This was also his chief complaint. Obviously, it would be difficult to test this problem if it were the only problem; however, it turned out that ultimately it was not his only sign of impending OBS. With more severe degrees of intellectual impairment, a general impoverishment of speech, and *slowing* of intellectual functions become apparent. For example, a person may correctly be able to subtract 7 from 100 serially, but do it with extreme slowness which can indicate difficulty in holding the question number and the answer number in his head simultaneously. This can also be a problem in memory, i.e., finding it difficult to remember the numbers to be subtracted.

Intellectual impairment is sometimes difficult to separate from memory impairment and sometimes requires formal testing to establish its presence.

LABILITY OF AFFECT

The first noticeable signs of lability of affect, which is *very* characteristic of organic brain syndromes, is inability to prevent exaggerated emotional responses. For example, the patient or his relatives may complain that he becomes overinvolved with television programs and laughs too hard or cries at the "drop of a hat" at any program. He may become outraged at small annoyances, an uncharacteristic action, and just as suddenly, forgive the annoyance and burst into tears of love for the persons receiving the forgiveness. Later he will show general impoverishment of emotional response, in that, things which previously would cause a response in him, no longer do so, unless it is an exaggerated one where he cannot control the emotional tone. Whatever personality characteristics a patient had beforehand, now also take on an exaggerated quality. He may become paranoid, more obsessive, or more negativistic. In general, the less likeable qualities of our personalities come into the fore when we begin to get "organic."

DELIRIUM AND DEMENTIA

What has just been described as the organic brain syndrome namely deficits in memory, orientation, intellect, judgment and affect occur in two forms—one, acute delirium which has other hallmarks such as hallucinations and occasionally delusions, and one chronic or progressive dementia where the prognosis is usually much less favorable and is considered permanent. Dementia may also be associated with hallucinations or delusions but is not of the same quality as delirium—as will be described.

Delirious patients manifest all the early signs noted for organic brain syndromes. They are disoriented usually only to time, although occasionally to place and person. Their recent memory is impaired far worse than their remote memory. Frequently they are hallucinating, primarily visually (visual hallucinations are more often associated with organic impairment than are auditory hallucinations), but if illicit drugs are producing the delirium then auditory hallucinations might also be present. Delirium is often directly attributable to drug, alcohol or suicidal ingestion of some poison such as an overdose of aspirin, or over-the-counter sleeping-pills, etc. Delirium occurs from many medical causes, from infection with or without fever to direct head injury. LSD sometimes causes delirium as do any other illicit drugs of that type or amphetamines. Early poisoning with barbiturates or heroin can cause disorientation and memory defects. As mentioned before schizophrenia itself can resemble a delirium. At any rate, the important thing is, if you have a patient with signs of delirium, you ascertain if there are immediate causes for it like head injury or drug ingestion, and refer the patient to an M.D. *immediately.*

Dementia (literally lack of mind) is what we commonly think of as senility. There can be many causes of it. If you know that the patient has a heart condition, his heart may not be pumping enough blood to his brain and may be responsible for the OBS you find on examination. Diabetes, for many reasons, can also be responsible for this condition, as can syphilis, kidney disorders, too few or too many salts in the blood, hardening of the arteries supplying the brain and thus decreasing the blood supply, etc. Your job is to find the signs of progressive cognitive, emotional, and intellectual deficit as has been described. It is difficult sometimes to pick these up in conversation. Towards the end of an interview, if I have reason to suspect organic impairment, and *even* if I *don't* have reason to suspect OBS, I tell the patient that I would like to test his memory and play a few mental games with him, no matter how silly the questions may seem. I then proceed to ask him several of the memory and orientation questions outlined in Chapter 6.

There are specific memory defects or other organic signs which go along with alcoholic brain disease. These will be described in the Chapter on Alcoholism.

CASE VIGNETTES OF PATIENT'S PAST
DRUG ABUSE

I have had several patients who have complained of specific difficulty with memory or concentration lasting years after the prolonged heavy ingestion of LSD, amphetamines or other drugs. I have had these patients tested, and the psychological tests could not pick up these so-called memory deficits. The patients describe it as "not being able to remember as fast as I used to be able to remember," "having difficulty remembering the common names for objects but being able to ultimately do so," and other subjective, internal, ideas that one's brain is not quite what it used to be. It is very difficult to separate the psychological reactions to heavy drug use and the possible but extremely subtle changes of mentation about which these patients complain. I have no doubt, that despite our inability to test these deficits with the finest psychological tools available, these changes in internal mental workings have taken place within the patient and he responds to them. These, untestable and undemonstrable "organic" complaints however, cannot presently be labeled as organic brain syndrome, although I fully expect that this will occur in the near future, as we further refine our psychological tools.

CHAPTER V

Is Your Patient Psychotic Due To Medical Disease?

According to the "Diagnostic and Statistical Manual" (DSM 11) of the American Psychiatric Association a person is psychotic "if their mental functioning is sufficiently impaired so as to interfere grossly with their capacity to meet the ordinary demands of life." This is a functional definition. Sometimes a person's ability to recognize reality and act appropriately with it is grossly lost. Reality-testing is the phrase used to describe the process of recognizing reality and acting in accordance with it. Other times a person's reality testing may be intact, in that they are aware of the realistic demands of life, but they are incapable of functioning to meet those demands. Severe functional disability is also included in this definition of psychosis.

A persons reality testing or functioning may be deficient because of hallucinations, delusions, severe mood disturbance, severe memory impairment, etc. On the other hand a person can be schizophrenic and not be psychotic by this definition.

The signs and symptoms of psychosis are generally agreed to be 1) hallucinations, 2) delusions, 3) profound depression or mania with or without hallucinations or delusions if the mood disorder prevents functioning in everyday life. Other symptoms such as "thought disorder" and specific types of delusions (e.g., paranoid) classify the psychoses into such categories as paranoid schizophrenia, psychotic depressive reaction, etc, depending on the associated symptoms, age of onset, previous episodes, relationship to drugs, etc.

In this chapter we will be concentrating on psychoses that have an origin in medical disease of which you can get hints if you ask the right questions.

It is important to note that the majority of the psychoses in this chapter are *also* associated with an organic brain syndrome. *Whenever* you feel a patient is psychotic and the patient has signs of organic brain syndrome as well, he must be seen by a psychiatrist or internist before embarking on psychotherapy. It is advisable to remember however, that acute schizophrenia can often be associated with confusion, clouded consciousness, disorientation, and memory or concentration defects and can, therefore, resemble an organic brain syndrome. It is precisely because this is true that at some point an M.D. should interview the patient so as to avoid treating hyperthyroidism with psychosis as schizophrenia, for example.

A good history can begin the differentiation between medical diseases causing the psychosis and the so-called functional psychoses, if you ask the right questions and do a good mental status examination (see Chapter 6). Probably the first question that should be asked upon initial contact with a psychotic patient should be "what drugs or alcohol has the patient been consuming?"

There are several syndromes of psychosis associated with alcohol and these are covered in the chapter on alcohol (Chapter 12). It is common knowledge that LSD, mescaline, amphetamines, barbiturates, or other illicit drugs, including marijuana, can cause psychosis which is difficult to differentiate from schizophrenia on occasion. Most of these "toxic" psychoses are associated with the signs of organic brain syndrome which were presented in Chapter 4, whereas as often as not an acute schizophrenic can still be oriented to time, place, and person and may even be able to do serial sevens (see Chapter 6).

A word here about the symptoms of psychosis. Visual hallucinations are more often seen in "organic" psychosis than are auditory hallucinations. This is quite important to remember. If a patient complains primarily of visual hallucinations one should be quite suspicious of organic psychosis. Although this is less true if the visual hallucinations are accompanied by auditory ones, it is still a cue to think "organic."

There are "normal" hallucinations called "hypnagogic hallucinations" which occur to some persons just before falling asleep. These are not considered psychotic if the rest of the mental status is clear. Particularly in older age groups however, confusion, disorientation and possibly hallucinations occur towards evening and/or a bedtime. This is characteristic of the onset of senile brain disease, more rightly entitled senile organic brain syndrome or senile dementia, and learning from the history of these symptoms should stimulate suspicion. Note that the hallucinations if present are usually visual and are almost always associated with confusion, memory impairment, and disorientation occurring in late evening and usually clearing by morning or early in the day. Often these symptoms can be managed by *small* doses of phenothiazines in late afternoon, and by that approach, hospitalization may possibly be avoided. It is also noteworthy that *large* doses of phenothiazines might make organic impairment worse. Small doses of phenothiazines are equivalent to 50 mg. of chlorpromazine (Thorazine) or less per day (see Chapter 8).

The symptoms of senile OBS as just described can be caused by anything which prevents blood from reaching the brain. This is generally called cerebral ischemia. As a result, loss of neurons or impairment of their transmission of impulses can occur. This can be due to cardiac conditions or general arteriosclerosis (hardening of the arteries) of the arteries to the brain, or of the smaller arteries and capillaries within the brain. *Whenever* you find psychosis *for the first time* in a patient over 50 think "organic." Very often, patients close to or over 50 will be depressed as well as psychotic since that is often the age of onset for psychotic depressive reaction and involutional melancholia. It is therefore imperative that you do a good mental status examination with all patients in older age groups (this does not mean that younger patients should be slighted).

CUSHINGS SYNDROME

Once in a while you may come across a person with this disease who is psychotic. Visual inspection of the patient is the best guide in this case. Cushings syndrome is a disease of the adrenal glands in which those glands produce too much cortisone. *The same symptoms can occur if your patient is taking cortisone for some other ailment.*

The patient is usually fat, with a heavy round face which is often excessively red. There may be profound depression associated with psychosis but mania is known to occur as well. Women tend to get more hair on their face and abdomen. You can ask the patient if they have noticed increased facial hair, increased weight, a tendency to drink a lot of water as well as urinate excessively. Frank diabetes is often also associated with this disease in which there is increased appetite as well as increased thirst. Frequently these symptoms occur in another disease of the adrenal glands, adreno-genital syndrome. The really important thing to remember is to LOOK at the patient and be suspicious if there is psychosis in a woman whose periods have stopped or become irregular, or in a man who recently developed a large paunch and is *heavy* especially on his (or her for that matter) upper back. The thickening of the fat pads on the nape of the neck and between the shoulder blades is the so-called "buffalo hump" which is characteristic of this disease. As noted, this can occur from cortisone pills being taken for some other disorder as well. It cannot be overemphasized, therefore, that a good medication history be obtained from the patient.

HYPERTHYROIDISM (OVERACTIVITY OF THE THYROID GLAND)

Interestingly, hyperthyroidism (whose anxiety attack-like symptoms were described in Chapter 1) is often associated with severe depression and/or psychosis. It is very important to distinguish this psychosis or depression from psychological or so-called functional psychoses, because it is entirely reversible with proper thyroid medications.

The patient will seem exceptionally nervous, sweating, subjectively complain of being too warm; he will also have a rapid heart rate or complain of palpitations; he may complain of insomnia. He will also have lost weight even in the face of increased appetite: the crucial question to be asked is—"have you lost or gained weight and how is your appetite?" Unfortunately, the most careful questioning will not differentiate hyperthyroidism from other nonmedically caused psychoses. The important thing is to be suspicious and OBSERVE the patient for signs like "bulging eyes," enlargement of the base of the neck in front, tremors, etc., and *ask* about excessive anxiety, sweating, palpitations, insomnia, etc.

Sometimes hyperthyroidism can resemble schizophrenia so that questions about eating, sleeping, and tremulousness are very important although they can not make the differentiation for you. The only sure way is to tell the supervising M.D. that hyperthyroidism is suspected and that he should order the proper laboratory blood tests.

It is important to recall that *this* psychosis may often be, but also may not be, associated with organic symptoms such as memory impairment, disorientation, and confusion.

HYPOTHYROIDISM

As noted in the preceding pages, diseases of the thyroid are prominent among causes for several psychiatric syndromes. It would probably be ideal for every patient who comes to a psychotherapist to have a battery of blood tests, including those for thyroid disease. Since this is not possible, clinical observations and suspicions will determine who is selected to have such tests.

Patients with hypothyroidism (underactivity of the thyroid gland) also develop psychoses with hallucinations and delusions, and these are usually associated with signs of organic brain syndrome, like memory defects. The patient may complain of, or you may notice, slowness of thought processes, depression, irritability, intolerance to cold, and general mental dullness or apathy. Depression and paranoid symptoms are commonly observed, but the personality structure of the person before the onset of the disease (premorbid personality structure) for the most part determines the symptoms within the psychosis.

A patient with hypothyroidism has been described earlier in the text. It will be recalled that patients with this disease have usually gained considerable amounts of weight depending on how long the hypothyroidism has been present. Their voice may be unusually low if female or have become lower if male or they may tell you that they have been hoarse for a few months and blame it on cigarettes. Their hair may have become coarse and dry and they may have lost some hair on their eyebrows, legs and abdomen or pubic region. Again, careful observation and questioning are what will prevent this patient from being treated for psychotic depressive reaction instead of hypothyroidism.

VITAMIN DEFICIENCIES OR EXCESSES

Deficiencies in vitamins particularly of the B variety can also be causes for organic brain syndrome with psychosis. Excess of vitamin D is another possible cause for psychosis, usually associated with OBS. The mechanisms by which vitamin deficiencies and excesses can cause psychosis with or without OBS are very complex. The important thing to remember is to ask the patient about his dietary habits and vitamin intake.

The list of possible medical diseases causing psychosis is very extensive and the preceding paragraphs list but a few examples. It would be very nice if all psychotic patients with or without OBS could have a complete medical and neurologic workup.

NEUROLOGIC DISEASES

In general, organic and psychological symptoms are frequent accompaniments to neurologic disease. Often the first sign of a brain tumor or minor stroke is a not-easily-definable "change in personality," most often noticed by relatives of the patient. A "simple" symptom such as fatigability can very occasionally herald myasthenia gravis. Euphoria is well known in acute multiple sclerosis, but depression and irritability are also common. Interestingly, in multiple sclerosis, lability of affect with some involuntary crying or laughter occurs but only after neurologic symptoms have emerged. It is not our purpose here to go into all neurologic diseases, but rather to point out the large overlap in symptomatology between neurologic and psychiatric diseases.

In general, when neurologic illnesses are associated with psychosis they are also associated with signs of organic brain syndrome. Sometimes psychotic patients can exhibit signs of apparent neurologic disease, especially when they show organic symptoms. I have had several patients who had severe depression, almost to the point where they couldn't talk. They could not function in their daily activities, and so in that aspect they were psychotic. They complained of poor memory, and indeed had very poor recent memory, to which their families attested. One of them had tremors as well, and we were sure he had an undisclosed neurological illness. None were disoriented, but on gross mental status testing all were deficient in some aspects, most generally associated with intellectual functioning. Complete neurologic workup, including arterial visualization in some, revealed no demonstrable neurologic problem. Then, and only then, when the neurologic workup was complete, we started them on antidepressants. As the depression lifted, so did the "organicity," until when the depression was gone, so were all the signs of organic brain syndrome, and, incidentally, tremors. On the other hand I had one patient with severe Parkinson's disease, whose tremors got progressively worse, who, although he didn't complain of depression, had all the psychomotor and vegetative signs of depression. Treatment of his depression with ECT resulted in a very significant decrease in the neurologic signs of his Parkinson's Disease. Improvement in Parkinsonian symptoms following ECT treatment of depression has also been reported in the literature. (Lebensohn and Jenkins, 1975).

CHAPTER VI

Outline Guide For First Interview

The circumstances surrounding the initial interview will determine its length and, hence, to what extent you will want to get all the information cited below in one session. For example, the patient's state of mind, to a certain extent, determines how long an interview he can tolerate, as well as what information you need. Other factors affecting this information gathering are: 1) whether you are or someone else is going to be the patient's primary therapist; 2) whether the patient is *in* the hospital or this interview might be determining if the patient needs hospitalization; 3) what your functional role is with the patient; 4) who is supervising you on the case or the interview, if anyone.

There are basically three main objectives in the first interview.

The first is to ascertain the person's "*chief complaint.*" That is, the reason that the patient gives for being at the interview. As the person talks and the *history* of the "chief complaint" becomes known, the next task is to arrive at a tentative working diagnosis, even if its "probably neurotic" or "probably psychotic". The third objective is to then decide what you are going to do about the situation, i.e., formulate a tentative working treatment plan. Sometimes all you have time for in this first session is to obtain the chief complaint and the history of the chief complaint, without being able to ask all the other important questions which are covered below. There are certain questions which really *must* be covered and others which can really be asked at a future time.

The first important thing is that you conceptualize the *PATIENT'S* view of why he came to see you. No matter how sophisticated your insight into his "*real*" problem may be, you might not want to immediately tell a patient who came to see you under pressure from his spouse, that the only thing that will save the marriage is a five times a week psychoanalysis. On the other hand, a psychotic patient who came under pressure from his family, and says he doesn't think there is anything wrong with him, can be told that you think that he has problems in certain areas (name them) and that he could be helped by both medication and psychotherapy if he was willing to give them a chance (either in or out of the hospital based on other factors defined below).

Remember, for the first interview you have three major tasks and that's *all*: ascertain the chief complaint, decide on a working diagnosis, and formulate what you are going to do about it. Don't let yourself get sidetracked by the patient into talking about his childhood, etc., and thus lose time during which you could be finding out about medical or biological signs which point to important diagnostic categories. If you are going to see the patient again you can talk about his childhood some other time; if you are *not* going to see him again, the discussion is irrelevant. Intrinsically there *is* nothing in this interview which precludes psychoanalytic therapy once the desirability of it is established and medication-responsive syndromes are ruled out. The outline below is a useful thing to have in mind as you interview the patient. It really contains the bare essentials that are necessary to achieving the three objectives stated above.

CHIEF COMPLAINT AND HISTORY OF CHIEF COMPLAINT

1. What is "Chief Complaint"?
2. *When* did "chief complaint" start?
3. *Why* did patient chose *this* day to seek help?
4. Did "chief complaint" ever occur in past and if so what set it off? How long did it last, what was treatment, did treatment work? How about self-treatment (medicines or drugs)?
5. MEDICATIONS, SELF-MEDICATIONS, past and present, don't forget BIRTH CONTROL PILLS.
6. DRUG USE OR ABUSE, past and present. Ask about: Hallucinations with or without drugs or alcohol.
7. ALCOHOL USE OR ABUSE, past and present. Ask about : Hallucinations with or without alcohol.
8. MEDICAL ILLNESSES PAST AND PRESENT, injuries, operations.
9. LOST OR GAINED WEIGHT during this *present* "chief complaint" or illness—how is appetite and taste of food?
10. How is patient *sleeping* these nights? How many hours? Does he wake up early, wake up intermittently, have difficulty falling asleep or not sleep, does he sleep during the day?
11. WHATEVER the chief complaint is, *always* ask patient if he has ever attempted suicide or has been thinking about it lately.
12. Ask about *Unusual Perceptual Phenomena.*
    Type Question: Have you ever experienced unusual things like hearing noises or voices that really weren't there? (checks both for psychosis and anything from a middle ear infection to a brain tumor). *Visual Hallucinations* in the *absence of any other signs* of psychosis or alcoholism should alert you to the possibility of organic brain impairment (diabetes, ischemia, tumor, etc.)
    Type Question: Have you ever had spots before your eyes or seen lights flashing when there were no real lights flashing? Have you ever had visions of people or animals?
    Type Question for other sensory phenomena: Have you ever *smelled* something funny that the people you were with didn't smell. (This question is particularly important to ask of persons who have violent outbursts of rage or rampages of impulsive behavior which last from minutes to hours—if validated by

EEG—these patients are said to have "uncinate fits" or temporal lobe epilepsy.) The nerves from the olfactory (smell) endings have connections in the temporal lobe and often people with this type of epilepsy smell "something burning" or some other description just before the attack occurs. Olfactory hallucinations also occur in schizophrenia.

If at this point you are out of time or the patient is emotionally fatigued, the following questions should be asked the next session. THESE QUESTIONS ARE ESSENTIAL and should be asked soon after beginning hospitalization or outpatient therapy since, as will be noted below, they are screening questions for various physical diseases which can mascarade as anything from schizophrenia to anxiety neurosis.

1. Change in Physical Appearance; Hair Distribution or Quantity. Enlargement of hat size, jaw, shoe size or glove size can point to acromegaly—a disorder of the pituitary gland. Changes in hair distribution can point to many things: loss of hair on legs and eyebrows—thyroid; increased abdominal hair and change in its pattern in females—adrenals, ovaries, pituitary, thyroid; loss of chest hair, facial hair in males—testicles, adrenals, pituitary.

2. Change in Voice: Males 12-16 Normal Deepening. Either sex's voice deepening after puberty could indicate thyroid problems, various neurologic disorders such as myasthenia gravis, or lung cancer in smokers. Incidently lung cancers are notorious for producing all kinds of chemicals and syndromes including psychosis.

3. Change in Menstrual Regularity. A host of things affect menstruation. It should be noted that phenothiazines, depression, tricyclics, anorexia nervosa, schizophrenia, and many other drugs and syndromes can be associated with complete cessation of menstruation. Mental state during pregnancy? The answer to this question may indicate whether presently used birth control pills are partly responsible for present condition.

4. Head injury or Seizure. Self-explanatory.

5. Fainting or Blackouts. Checks for anemia, hypoglycemia, hysteria, hyperventilation, orthostatic hypotension, petit mal epilepsy, alcoholism and many other causes for brain impairment.

6. *Is Patient a Food-Faddist or Vitamin Taker.* People on high protein, low calorie diets who eat fish in excess of what the programs recommend, or other fish-eaters have occasionally been found to have mercury poisoning in the United States (many more in Japan and other countries whose main source of animal protein is fish), which presents itself as nervousness, irritability, etc., and can be confused with neurotic symptoms. Vitamin faddists can get vitamin poisoning—particularly vitamins A and D both of which can present psychiatrically.

7. *Memory and Concentration.* These can be disrupted both by psychological disease and organic brain disease and are crucial in diagnosing organic brain disease. It is common for acute schizophrenics to be unable to perform the memory and concentration tests on the mental status examination. However, when they are calmed and improved some weeks later, they are quite able to do so. Persons with permanent organic brain impairment with psychosis may be "cured" of their psychosis, but they remain unable to recall what they had for dinner the night before, etc. by the mental status examination.

FORMAL MENTAL STATUS

1. Orientation Tests
(a) Time: what is today's date; month, day, year?
(b) Place: what is the name of this place; what place did you come from?
(c) Person: who am *I*? (Don't ask the patient who *he* is unless you suspect hysterical (fake) amnesia; no matter how "organic" somebody gets, they *almost never* forget their name; hysterics however, *will* sometimes deny that they remember their name.) The patient may not be able to recall your name but should be able to say that you are the nurse, the doctor, the social worker, etc.
1. Have we ever met before? (This checks for confabulation, a specific defect in which the patient, being aware of "holes" in his

memory attempts to fill in the gaps with stories he is not quite sure did not happen. Confabulation is seen in alcoholic brain damage more often than in senile or other organicities.)

2. Memory Tests. (a) Recent Memory: What did you have for your most recent meal?; What did you have for the meal before that?

1. I am going to tell you three unrelated words; I want you to try to remember them. I will ask you what they are later. Tennis, cereal, blue, repeat once and have the patient repeat them (also tests concentration).

(b) Remote Memory and Concentration—Serial 7's: Tell the patient to subtract 7 from 100 then 7 from that and 7 from that, continue even if they are doing it totally wrong, until you have decided, based on either their intellectual or educational level or their organic brain impairment that they are incapable of doing this (or capable of it).

With patients whom I presume to be well educated, I often tell them that I wish to check their memory, and I ask them if they remember their algebra. I then ask them a simple equation in algebra and if they can answer it I presume this particular part of the mental status examination to be okay. If they can't do the algebra I proceed to 100 minus 17 and 98 plus 19, and then finally to 100 minus 7. This way of proceeding tests educational level and memory function and can give many valuable clues.

(c) Who is the President of the U.S. now? Who was the President before him? and before him? Most organically *unim*paired people can name the presidents backwards in sequence for about five presidents if they are old enough, or have completed high school. Uneducated, or very unintelligent people may only be able to name two. Organically impaired persons may recall those 30 years previous, but be unable to name recent ones.

3. Proverbs. Although this is part of the "mental status" examination it is highly debated as to *what* if anything, proverb testing measures. Supposedly, if the person answers in certain ways it may either be, self-referential or be indicative of "concreteness" which allegedly occurs more often in schizophrenia and in some organic brain syndromes. Examples will follow. Proverbs may not be too useful diagnostically if the patient has never heard them before or was not brought up in this country. It can be argued that adults of normal intelligence should be able to get the abstract meaning of the proverb even if they never heard it before. However, *in the presence of an otherwise clear mental status*, I personally would draw no conclusions if the patient could not abstract the proverbs.

Ask the patient what does this proverb mean? Have you ever heard it before?

1. People who live in glass houses shouldn't throw stones. The standard answers to this should include the idea of either those who are equally guilty shouldn't point fingers at others or those who are equally vulnerable or open to criticism shouldn't criticize others.

The "concrete" answer classically is "because they'll break the windows" followed by an *inability* to give the other (more abstract) meanings.

2. A stitch in time saves nine. Standard answer includes concept of catching trouble early, or doing some task before it gets too big or out of hand. I had a schizophrenic patient who said "well, if I sew it up I only use nine stitches and I save time. I saved nine dollars by stitching nine times." This is, you will admit, both concrete (*not abstract*) and self-referential, besides not making too much sense.

You can use any proverbs you know and the patient says he has heard before. You can even ask if the person remembers whether they *ever* knew what the proverb meant. Inability to abstract on proverbs however, by *itself*, is *not diagnostic* of anything.

BACK TO RECENT MEMORY AND CONCENTRATION

Do you recall the three words I told you to memorize: What were they? Tennis, cereal, and blue.

It is not necessary to ask the above questions like a Gestapo agent, they can be interspersed into the conversation between you and the patient. Here is an example of how it can be done.

T = Therapist, P = Patient.

T: "What made you come here today?"

P: "My nerves have been getting progressively worse."

T: "Since when?"

P: "Well, my mother died three years ago and I haven't been the same since. I've been nervous and irritable and depressed."

T: (Checking for family history of suicide) "What did your mother die of?"

P: "Chirrhosis of the liver and pancreatitis."

T: "Oh was she an alcoholic?" (T's thoughts—probable family history of depression since most alcoholics, especially female alcoholics are chronically depressed.)

P: "Yes, she was alcoholic and I never had a father. She made my nerves worse when she was alive. She made my father's nerves bad too, which is probably why he divorced her. I was only 3 when they separated. She was drinking heavily even at that time."

T: "What do you mean when you say your nerves are bad?"

P: "I've been hearing strange things like people knocking on doors, but I go to the door and there's no one there. . . . And I can't concentrate and I think I'm losing my memory. I can't remember the simplest things."

T: "Have you been using any drugs?" (note signs of possible organic brain disorder—memory defects, concentration, irritability).

P: "I used to use a lot of "speed" when I was depressed in the past, but I haven't used anything except "pot" lately."

T: "When was the last time you used "speed?"

P: "Oh about two months ago, I've been trying to diet."

T: "How long have you been depressed?"

P: "I've been depressed for three years since my mother died."

T: "Did your mother's death make you depressed?" (NEVER ASSUME!)

P: "I got depressed before her death actually because she was sick and she leaned on me a lot. My mother was really terrible—even when I was a child. She was always drunk, she beat me a lot, she never let me have boyfriends. When she got really sick from the alcoholism she wanted me to take total care of her. That's when I started to get depressed."

T: "Did you ever get depressed before that?" (Be wary of getting sidetracked about childhood.)

P: "I've been depressed my whole life it seems, but actually sometimes I'm normal, in fact sometimes I'm hyperactive."

T: "What do you mean by hyperactive?"

P: "Well, I clean the house, move furniture around, get interested in going back to school again, get interested in all kinds of projects."

T: "Do you get interested or do you actually do all kinds of projects?"

P: "I actually do some projects, especially those that I can finish fast. I do others when I'm really high."

T: "Too high or just normally feeling good."

P: "No, too high."

T: "What do you mean by too high?"

P: "Well, I'm feeling so good that I make everyone laugh around me. My thoughts speed up and I can't concentrate—and that's off "speed.""

P: "I don't like to sleep when I'm high either. I only get about four hours and that's enough. Sleeping seems like a waste of time when I feel that way."

T: "How are you sleeping now?"

P: "I can't sleep at night at all; every time I lie down I just think bad thoughts. I can't remember anything good about my mother, only the bad things, that's what I mean about my memory going bad."

T: "Are you sleeping during the day?"

P: "Yes, that's all I do is sleep and eat. I've gained 40 pounds in three years. I took off ten, but I'm still 30 pounds overweight."

T: "So you generally gain weight when you're depressed? What is it like when you're high?"

P: "I always go on a diet when I'm high."

T: "Do you lose weight?"

P: "Oh yes, I'm much fatter now than I usually am."

T: "How long do the highs last and how long do the downs last?"

P: "A few weeks for the highs and a few years for the downs."

T: "Have you ever tried to kill yourself?"

P: "I tried three times. Twice I took overdoses but I got scared and realized I really didn't want to die so I vomited up the pills. Last year I slit my wrist."

T: "Did you need stitches?"

P: "It was just a scratch, no stitches."

T: "So you get depressed enough to want to die but then you really don't want to."

P: "I was drunk both times I took the overdoses."

T: "Do you drink when you're depressed?"

P: "I drink about one drink and I'm drunk and angry and depressed and I black out and can't remember anything afterwards—I don't even remember taking the drink."

T: "Do you ever black out when you're not drinking?"

P: "No."

T: "You said you've tried to kill yourself in the past; have you thought about doing it recently?"

P: "I've thought about it but I'm not going to do it."

T: "Why not?"

P: "I can only get the courage when I'm drunk and my husband doesn't let me get drunk anymore."

T: "I'd like to get back to the 'knocks at the door'. Have you ever heard other things like clicks or actual voices when people were not around?"

P: "I heard like bells but I knew they weren't really there."

T: "Aside from blacking out after one drink, have you ever been unconscious or had a head injury?"

P: "I fell off a horse when I was about ten years old and my mother said I was unconscious for a few minutes but I don't remember anything about it."

T: "I'd like to go back to the original problem for a while. What made you come here *today* specifically?"

P: "Well, I just couldn't take it anymore; my nerves were driving me crazy. I want to get my head together . . . I am so nervous all the time and I'm horribly depressed."

T: "Have you taken any medicine for your nerves?"

P: "Yeah, the family doctor gave me little white tablets a long time ago, but I ran out of them about two months ago."

T: "You're not taking *anything* now—no medicines, no drugs, not anything?"

P: "Well not for the last two months anyway."

T: "How about birth control pills?"

P: "Oh, yes, of course I take those, but that's not medicine."

T: "Not in the usual sense, but birth control pills are depressing to some people. When did you start taking them?"

P: "About two years ago."

T: "You've been depressed for three years and off and on before that; did you ever see a psychiatrist for it?"

P: "Before my mother died she wouldn't let me, and since she died I figured I was just still mourning and no one could help me. My husband has been trying to help but he just makes me feel worse because I can't do the things a wife is supposed to do, so he does them and then I feel guilty. I can't even go to bed with him."

This is merely an excerpt from an interview, and obviously many things are not covered, particularly psychological issues around this patient's mother's death, and further probing about why the patient came that particular day—which may be because of her husband, another area which is not presented in the excerpt. What can be gleaned from this part of the interview is the patient's chief complaint, its partial history, her sleeping and eating habits, drug and alcohol usage, one important piece of family history, a smattering of checking for unusual perceptual phenomena and the recognition of what is *left out*, providing a concept of what *should be included* is kept in mind. One very important part of this interview which is not included is the formal mental status examination. This is particularly important since this woman was complaining of vaguely organic symptomatology. The mental status examination in this woman turned out to be normal. It was introduced to her by saying, "I want to check your memory and concentration. Some of the things I ask you will seem silly, but please go along with me anyway." Every therapist has his or her own way of introducing this vital part of the interview.

Chief complaint, as stated by patient, "nerves getting bad" as perceived by the therapist and patient (ultimately); depression three years or more duration.

DIAGNOSTIC POSSIBILITIES

1. a) Cyclothymic personality with hysterical features.

b) The possibility of manic-depressive illness should be kept in mind but needs more supporting evidence such as distinct phases obvious to husband and clearer definition of highs without the probable use of amphetamines.

2. Amphetamine-induced depression with incipient psychosis. Note: patient denies recent amphetamine abuse, but this should still be a consideration.

3. Possible pathological intoxication. (Pathological intoxication is the occurrence of hostile, violent or impulsive behavior, with intoxication, blackouts and memory loss for the period of time following one or at the most two normal size alcohol-containing drinks.) This patient attempted suicide twice after having one cocktail, which can be considered impulsive since she immediately aborted her own attempts.

TENTATIVE TREATMENT PLAN

1. Possibly hospitalize unless extreme objections from husband, for, despite denial, patient is probably suicidal although she is not likely to attempt suicide while sober. Possibility exists, however, that she will deliberately drink, knowing that she is likely to attempt suicide again.

Here again then, without additional commentary is the outline for the first interview.

Ascertain as much of the following information as possible.

CHIEF COMPLAINT—WHAT IS IT?

1. When did it start.
2. Why did patient choose *this* day to seek help.
3. History of chief complaint

(a) Has it occurred in past; if yes, when, how long did it last, what set it off, was it treated, if so, by whom or what and did treatment work.

4. What medicines or drugs is patient now using and has patient used for similar discomfort in past.

5. Drug abuse, particularly amphetamines and barbiturates and alcohol—in *all* age groups; younger patients should be asked about hallucinogens, marijuana, hashish, cocaine, etc.

6. Relevant medical illnesses, operations or injuries.

7. Biologic Signs

Sleep disorders: waking up much too early; inability to fall asleep; persistent intermittent awakening; too much sleep; inability to get out of bed (more than ten hours sleep); sleep during day; not sleeping at night.

Appetite disorders: eating excessively; being excessively *hungry* but *eating normally* for fear of gaining weight; loss of appetite; food being tasteless; WEIGHT GAIN or LOSS.

Psychomotor symptoms: *observe*: foot tapping, hand wringing or fist clenching; facial expression; *rate* of speech; use or nonuse of hands in talking; unusual body posture; static body position, restlessness.

8. Suicide potential *presently* as well as past attempts.

ADDITIONAL DIAGNOSTIC QUESTIONS NECESSARY TO TENTATIVE WORKING DIAGNOSIS:

1. unusual perceptual phenomena and hallucinations.
2. changes in physical appearance,
    especially: loss of hair on legs, eyebrows; pubic region, thinning of head-hair, excessive hair anywhere; enlargement of base of neck in front or in back; drooping of one eyelid or one corner of mouth.
3. changes of voice; slurring of speech.
4. changes in *memory, concentration*.
5. regularity of menstruation; mental state during pregnancies.
6. Sexual enjoyment.
7. head injury or seizure (convulsion).
8. fainting, blackouts.
9. concern for physical health; vitamin taking.
10. FORMAL MENTAL STATUS EXAMINATION especially

indicated where difficulties in memory and concentration are in question.

Should you feel it necessary, in order to set up your personal style with the patient, nothing prevents you from indicating that this style of questioning and interacting is really only for the first or second interview and that future sessions will more than likely be rather different.

CHAPTER VII

Minor Tranquilizers

The minor tranquilizers are called "minor" to distinguish them from the phenothiazines and phenothiazine-like drugs which are called major tranquilizers because they are usually used in more serious psychiatric disorders. The minor tranquilizers are used by themselves in neurotic disorders and *sometimes* in conjunction with major tranquilizers or antidepressants in more major psychiatric conditions like severe depressions or psychoses.

The minor tranquilizers discussed here are:

Librium	(chlordiazepoxide)	
Valium	(diazepam)	
Serax	(oxazepam)	
Meprotabs	(Meprobamate)	Solacen (tybamate)
Equanil	(Meprobamate)	
Meprospan	(Meprobamate)	
Miltown	(Meprobamate)	

There are many others listed in the Appendix under minor tranquilizers, but most of the studies of efficacy of minor tranquilizers versus placebo or versus each other have been done using the drugs listed above (Klein and Davis, 1969). They are very good antianxiety agents and some are good anticonvulsants. Librium, Valium, and Serax are very closely allied chemically. Equanil and Miltown, Meprospan, and Meprotabs are the same drug under four brand names, the latter two (Meprospan and Meprotabs) have a sustained release form. Other drugs, like Librax, have Librium combined with antispasmodic agents for the stomach, and Miltrate which has an antiangina drug in it. Dalmane is a sleeping pill, derived closely from Valium-type chemicals. In this chapter we will consider simply the minor tranquilizers as listed above and not deal with combination products or derivatives.

In talking about the minor tranquilizers it is necessary to immediately begin talking about dosage. In doses of less than 20 mg per day of Librium many studies show Librium equal to placebo (Klein and Davis, 1969). However, in *most* studies on neurotic anxiety, all the drugs listed and barbiturates in sedative doses were better than placebo when used in high enough dosage. Most studies showed that any of the tranquilizers listed above was equal to the effects of any other, if given in pharmacologically equivalent doses, to neurotic anxious patients with or without other symptoms such as depression or phobia. The majority of studies indicated that the minor tranquilizers were not as good as phenothiazines at relieving anxiety when used alone in major psychiatric illnesses such as schizophrenia.

As with any tranquilizer, including the major tranquilizers, the drugs under discussion can be depressing. Here, clinical judgment is very important. Anxiety itself is depressing and is often difficult to separate from depression clinically. In attempting to assess how depressed the patient is, versus how much his anxiety plays a role in his depression, I usually use biological criteria. If the patient has a sleep disorder such as early morning awakening, a loss of appetite or heavily increased appetite or other biologic signs mentioned in the chapter on depression, I usually assume the depression to be primary, and I treat it with antidepressants. If however, no biological signs of depression are present, but the patient complains of depression and anxiety, I usually assume the anxiety to be primary and treat it with minor tranquilizers. Often a combination of antidepressants (tricyclic type) and minor tranquilizers is useful even when no biological signs of depression exist. However as already noted, depressions without the biological signs are less likely to respond to the antidepressants. It is important to realize that minor depression, without biological signs, will probably respond most favorably to psychotherapy alone or psychotherapy combined with minor tranquilizers if the anxiety component is strong. Often, when anxiety is relieved the patient feels less depressed despite the fact that the tranquilizers can be psychologically depressing.

The minor tranquilizers are *not* placebo. They work, and work well, at relieving anxiety, tension, and associated mild depression, apathy, etc. which often result from anxiety.

The major problem with the *minor tranquilizers* is that they can be *physically addicting.* They are not really addicting in low doses but can be seriously addicting in high doses. They also show the typical course of any addicting drug which begins with tolerance. That is, the original dose of the drug no longer gives the original antianxiety response; more drug is needed to obtain the same response. It is important, therefore, to keep checking with the patient about the quantity of tranquilizer he is taking. There is a strong tendency to increase the dosage once the patient has found that the drug alleviates his symptoms. Doses of Librium or Valium in excess of 75 mg per day are probably addictive and should not be withdrawn abruptly. Doses of Meprobamate of above 8 capsules a day should be considered addictive and should not be withdrawn abruptly either.

The signs and symptoms of withdrawal from any of these drugs are similar to withdrawal of any central nervous system depressant. These are: excitability, nervousness, leg cramps and twitches, nausea and vomiting, and possibly convulsions *if* the addiction has existed for a long time and/or on a very high dose.

Interestingly enough, diazepam is now the drug of choice used by many physicians in the United States to stop epileptic seizures and prevent them in alcoholic withdrawal. It is a better choice than phenothiazines for epileptic patients since phenothiazines lower the threshold for seizure activity. As with any tranquilizer, major or minor, the effects of the drug are increased by, or are additive with, the effects of liquor, sleeping pills, anesthetics, and other tranquilizers. Patients should be warned about drinking while on the minor tranquilizers since they will tend to get sleepy more easily on their usual amount of liquor.

SIDE EFFECTS

There are extremely few consistent side effects from the minor tranquilizers. One has already been noted, namely, depression. Probably the most common side effect is drowsiness, which may wear off in three days if the dose is not too high. If drowsiness persists, the dose may have to be lowered. Other very infrequent reactions such as "paradoxical excitement," panic or rage do occur.

All in all, however, the minor tranquilizers are excellent drugs for the treatment of neurotic anxiety or mixed anxiety and depression, as well as for anxiety and tension resulting from physical illness. They can be taken with almost all other drugs without harmful effects. Caution with liquor and sleeping pills should be exercised. As with *any* drug, the possibility of deformed children should be kept in mind if the drugs are given during the first three months of pregnancy. It is always advisable to stop all medications if possible during pregnancy.

Often, I have seen schizophrenic patients who are taking major tranquilizers benefit from the addition of minor tranquilizers. This probably is due to the more antipsychotic properties of the phenothiazines as distinct from their antianxiety properties. The minor tranquilizers are specific antianxiety agents but have *no* antipsychotic properties. In other words, minor tranquilizers are *not a substitute* for phenothiazines and should not be used as such. They *may* help further reduce anxiety in patients who also need antipsychotic drugs as well.

The minor tranquilizers can often be used to calm agitation in unipolar depression as well. Unfortunately, however, this is not usually the case, and major tranquilizers are frequently needed in conjunction with tricyclic antidepressants. However, given the additive side effects of major tranquilizers and tricyclic antidepressants, it is worth a try to give the anxious depressed patient a fair trial on minor tranquilizers before going to the major ones.

A word about the use of minor tranquilizers in neurotic anxiety. It is a very critical decision to use minor tranquilizers in mild to moderate neurotic anxiety. There is certainly validity in the concept that if one chemically deprives the neurotic patient of the anxiety he is experiencing, he will be less likely to seek solutions to the conflicts which are presumably causing the anxiety. However, and this is why the decision is so crucial, anxiety in excess can itself interfere with psychotherapeutic work and the ability to deal effectively with interpretations.

In general, at least temporarily, minor tranquilizers are indicated if the person is dysfunctional in a major area of his life *as a result of neurotic anxiety.* Even this statement needs modification, however, because certainly phobias produce tremendous anxiety in the face of the phobic situation, yet reducing that anxiety will probably not reduce the phobia—even if the phobia is causing a major dysfunction. In short, minor tranquilizers do not always work. They reduce anxiety, not conflict. On the other hand, where neurotic anxiety is causing severe difficulty with work, relaxation, or interpersonal relations, minor tranquilizers can be of considerable benefit when used as a temporary measure.

CHAPTER VIII

Major Tranquilizers: Phenothiazines

Major Tranquilizers: Antipsychotic agents, Phenothiazines, Thioxanthines, Butyrophenones

Phenothiazines were discovered in the mid-1950's and to a great extent are responsible for shortening the duration of hospital stay for many types of psychotic patients. Some of the more commonly used phenothiazines are:

Thorazine (chlorpromazine)
Mellaril (thioridazine)
Stelazine (trifluoperazine)
Vesprin (trifluoperazine)
Serentil (mesoridazine)
Quide (Piperacetazine)

Prolixin (fluphenazine)
Permitil (fluphenazine)
Trilafon (perphenazine)
Compazine (prochlorperazine)
Phenergan (promethazine)
Sparine (promazine)
Tindal (acetophenazine)

A more complete list is found in the Appendix under major tran-quilizers. The following drugs, although not phenothiazines, have similar actions against psychotic thinking and agitation and have similar side effects (in talking about phenothiazines these drugs are *understood to be included*):

Haldol (haloperidol)	Taractan (chloroprothixene)
	Navane (thiothixene)
Serenace (haloperidol)	Solatran (chloroprothixene)

Phenothiazines are also potent antiemetics (prevent nausea and vomiting) and some of them, like Compazine and Phenergan, are used more commonly for that purpose than for antipsychotic action.

Essentially, phenothiazines are used in treating psychotic thinking, (thought disorganization and delusions) as well as hal-lucinatory experience and agitation. They can be and are some-times used in severe neurotic anxiety states. They are used to control acute mania, because the specific drug for mania, namely Lithium, takes about two weeks to exert its maximum antimanic effect whereas phenothiazines act within hours if a high enough dose is given. Clearly, the phenothiazines are used in a wide variety of conditions but mainly where there exists psychosis with or without agitation or severe agitation even if unaccompanied by psychosis. They used to be used for alcoholic hallucinosis and "D.T's" but diazepam (Valium) and chlordiazepoxide (Librium) have been found to be more advantageous for alcoholic states since they also help prevent withdrawal seizures.

The dosage of phenothiazines is extremely variable and does not depend solely on either the size or weight of the patient nor his state of psychotic disorganization or agitation. This is important to realize because often, unconsciously, we tend to feel differently about patients whom we know are on supposedly large doses of phenothiazines. Studies have been reported (Klein and Davis, 1969) that chlorpromazine (Thorazine) in doses at or below 300 mg/day is equal to or slightly better than placebo *as often* as it is found to be more effective than placebo. However, when given at doses of 500 mg/day or more it was always more effective than placebo. The list of dosages of other antipsychotic drugs which are equivalent to 100 mg of chlorpromazine is very extensive. The prescribing physician should be consulted for an idea of the approximate equivalent to chlorpromazine of the antipsychotic agent the patient is taking.

Side effects are often dose-dependent; that is, reducing the dose may reduce the side effects. Allergic reactions such as jaundice (hepatitis) or skin reactions such as rashes or swelling, redness and itching upon exposure to sunlight are generally *not* dose-dependent and can even occur occasionally with one dose.

Generally, although not being the prescriber of these drugs, you will usually be in the position to observe their side effects as well as their main effect. The main effects of phenothiazines and similar drugs are: 1) elimination of hallucinations; 2) decrease in delusional thinking; 3) decrease in agitation; 4) organization of thought processes and verbal productions; 5) decrease in anxiety. A comment here. The patient may still have delusions, but he no longer "cares" about them as much.

It is important to realize that improvement in these parameters is dependent on many factors, such as route of administration for example. Agitation can be eliminated almost immediately by giving enough phenothiazine I.M. (injected into the muscle). This usually puts the patient to sleep temporarily, but the delusions and hallucinations will take much longer to disappear—around 1-2 weeks if the proper dose is administered over that period of time. Should the patient continue to hallucinate or be heavily delusional after 2 weeks on a particular dose, you should suggest to your medical back-up that the dose be increased.

The most commonly seen side effect is "sedation." The patient will complain of feeling sleepy. This is more true of certain types of phenothiazines than with others, but *all* can and *do* cause sedation. You can reassure the patient that the sleepiness is a side effect and will wear off in a week or so. If the patient still feels sleepy or "stoned" after 14 days on a drug, a decreased dose may be considered. This is also important to note after a patient has been on the same dose for 6 to 8 months. If at that time he begins to feel sleepy and it is *certain* that it is phenothiazine related, it may indicate that he is improving and also needs a slight decrease in dose.

You will often be asked if other preparations or drugs can be used safely with phenothiazines. In general, most over-the-counter preparations are safe with phenothiazines. The big caution is *alcohol* which makes the person on phenothiazines very sleepy very quickly if he attempts to drink as much as he did without phenothiazines. Also, some over-the-counter cough medications contain narcotics or synthetic-narcotic-like drugs which also add to the sedative properties of the phenothiazines. Naturally, sleeping pills of any type, nonprescription included, are additive with these drugs. In general however, the phenothiazines are "safe" drugs to take with most other drugs. This is definitely opposite to the case of MAO inhibitors which will be discussed shortly.

The next most common side effects that patients complain of are dry mouth, stuffy nose and constipation, all of which are due to the anticholinergic properties of phenothiazines. These side effects generally persist as long as the drug is taken. I usually suggest that the patient chew sugarless* gum for the dry mouth and take an occasional tablespoonful of milk of magnesia if the constipation gets too bad. Less commonly, patients on phenothiazines will complain of blurred vision at close range. Sometimes a different phenothiazine is worth a try in this case, if it does as good a job as the original in checking the symptomatology which necessitated phenothiazines. Otherwise a simple pair of over-the-counter magnifying glasses often alleviates the difficulty. If the dose is high enough (more than 200 mg of chlorpromazine or the equivalent per day) almost every patient will experience orthostatic hypotension (ortho=change in; static=position; hypo=low; tension=blood pressure). In other words, when going from lying down or sitting, to standing or walking, the patient will experience the sensation of blood rushing to or from his head (sufficient quantity is actually not being pumped up to his head) due to the fact that his blood pressure drops slightly when he changes his position. The body rapidly accommodates this condition and soon the sensation of dizziness or light-headedness has past. He can then go on about his business, since his blood pressure does not usually stay too low. He may feel his heart beat faster or pound just after the head sensation and this is one of the ways the body

*The sugarless part is very important to prevent mouth infections which result from mouth breathing and bacteria which grow in sugar. (They mouth-breathe because their nose is stuffed.)

increases the blood to the head. There is little danger if he is told to change positions *slowly* and to stand for 30 seconds before beginning to walk, after rising from lying to sitting. Unlike sedation this side effect continues as long as the drug is taken.

The following side effects are the ones most talked about and overrated in terms of frequency; these are, Parkinsonian side effects. "Parkinsonian" refers to the fact that many of the reactions to be described are seen in Parkinson's disease which is a complex disorder of certain nerve-cell bodies in the brain. It suffices to say that phenothiazines are thought to cause similar but only temporary disorders in those same brain centers and, hence, cause the side effects seen. (For a fuller understanding see Chapter 13).

Some of the Parkinsonian side effects are:

(1) a "pill-rolling" motion made with one or both hands individually where the thumb is repeatedly and rhythmically moved back and forth across the semiclosed fingers as if the person were dealing cards or rolling pills in his hand. This stops if the hand is used but will begin, involuntarily, again, if the hand is not being used.

(2) a rigid way of walking—rigid gait—where the person looks sort of stiff and may not lift his feet off the floor as before. This is mockingly referred to by chronic knowledgeable patients as the "Thorazine shuffle." It can be reduced considerably by the addition of anti-Parkinsonian drugs (these will be taken up shortly).

(3) akathisia—not true Parkinsonism but commonly seen in side reactions to phenothiazines. This is motor restlessness, an inability to sit still, constant nonrhythmic motion of hands and feet, and subjective complaints such as "can't sit still," "want to move all the time," etc. This is probably *the* one most difficult side effect since it can be *misinterpreted* as indicating increasing anxiety and *more* phenothiazine will be *mistakenly* given. Since anti-Parkinson agents do not usually reduce this symptom, the drug dosage must be reduced or a different phenothiazine tried. Obviously, reducing the dosage may cause a recurrence of psychotic symptoms which *can* be differentiated from the motor restlessness caused by the drug, but this is a very tricky decision sometimes.

Another almost universally complained of side effect is weight gain. It is really uncertain yet whether phenothiazines merely increase appetite or if they cause increased accumulation of fat tis-

sue in some metabolic way. In any case, this can become a significant problem with many patients who discover this and then refuse to take the medicine. However weight gain can be prevented
if caloric intake is reduced. Some anti-Parkinsonian agents commonly used are:

Artane (trihexiphenidyl)   Kemadrin (procyclidine)
Akineton (biperiden)   Cogentin (benztropine mesylate)

These drugs were originally used for Parkinson's disease itself until
L-DOPA supplanted them. L-DOPA is not a good drug to use
against the side effects of phenothiazines because in various people
it induces mood altering effects or other psychological effects
which are not beneficial to the person in need of phenothiazines.
Unfortunately, the most disturbing side-effects of phenothiazines
are not really altered much by the anti-Parkinsonian drugs. That
is, blurred vision, weight gain, and akathisia are not usually affected by these agents. However, the tremor of hands, "pill-
rolling," rigidity, shuffling gait, etc. can be alleviated with these
agents and they are often worth a try. Many M.D.s prescribe these
prophylactically with the phenothiazines. This is both unneces-
sary, since susceptible side effects only occur about 5-10% of the
time, and unwise, since these agents also *cause* dry mouth, blurred
vision, and constipation.

There are some really rare side effects of which you should be
aware in case they happen to one of your patients.

In *either* males or females, breast enlargement and/or lactation
may occur (milk or fluid from breasts). Females on high doses of
phenothiazines may not menstruate for long periods of time. As
was mentioned in Chapter 2, men may have no emission of fluid
during ejaculation but have no trouble having orgasm (psychosexual pleasure as opposed to physiologic emission). Another occasional side effect of phenothiazines and similar drugs is a severe
decrease in, or elimination of, a certain type of white blood cell.
These white blood cells are essential to the body in preventing infection; they are called granulocytes and the absence of them in
the blood is called agranulocytosis and is potentially fatal. This
usually begins as a sore throat and "swollen glands" (under the
jaw). There is usually a fever and other symptoms and signs of in-

fection. About 90% of the cases of agranulocytosis occur in the first eight weeks of treatment. (Shader and Dimascio, 1970). Therefore be *especially* alert for complaints of sore throat, "head cold," etc. during this period. Send the patient immediately to a doctor. If sore throat, and related symptoms occur at anytime during phenothiazine treatment, it is worth while getting the patient to a doctor for examination and a "blood count."

There are two other rare side effects you may see. Both involve the muscles of the jaw, tongue, and face. These are the acute buccolingual dystonias and tardive dyskinesias. Acute dystonia usually occurs at the beginning of treatment with phenothiazines or the other antipsychotics. It may occur even after one dose. The reaction may also involve the muscles of the neck as well as face. There may be torticollis—a condition where the neck muscles twist the head around and down with the ear close to the shoulder. Abnormal contraction of the face muscles causes a severely contorted (sometimes one-sided contortion) facial expression. Another type of acute dystonic reaction involving the tongue, causes it to swell up and be involuntarily protruded. This is sometimes accompanied by involuntary chewing motions of the jaws. Both acute dystonic reactions can be considerably alleviated by anti-Parkinsonian drugs and antihistamines, both usually given I.M. All three chemical classes of antipsychotic drugs presently on the U.S. market are capable of producing this reaction.

The other rare reaction occurs only after very prolonged, moderately high dose administration of anti-psychotic drugs. This is tardive dyskinesia. In this reaction the muscles of the jaw, mouth, and tongue combine to produce involuntary chewing motions, lip smacking motions and generalized contortions of the parts named. It should be emphasized that these rare reactions are truly *rare* and should not curtail the treatment of someone who is in need of antipsychotic medication.

CHAPTER IX

Antidepressants

There are two basic categories of antidepressants, the tricyclic and the monoamine oxidase inhibitors (MAOIs). The theory behind the actions of these drugs is the most developed of any of the biochemical theories we have in psychiatry to explain depression and its possible biochemical causes. (See Chapter 13.) It is vital for you to know however, that recent evidence suggests that, different types of depressions respond better either to tricyclics or MAOIs, but that there is also considerable overlap in response by the various depressions.

It is obvious from the outset, therefore, that a careful and thorough diagnosis and history be made before making any specific suggestion to one's medical back-up. (See Chapter 3 on Depression.) To reiterate very briefly what was said about depression, there are basically three types of depression: unipolar (which may be the first depression or recurrent depression with no history of hypomania), bipolar, and neurotic (or "reactive") depression. Unipolar and bipolar may exist with or without psychosis and almost always have consistent sleep and appetite disorders associated with them. Neurotic-reactive depression may be a chronic lifelong characterologic state or a brief episode in re-action to some life experience. In general neurotic-reactive depressions are not associated with biological signs and MAY NOT RESPOND to either type of antidepressant. Difficulty falling asleep *may* be common in neurotic depression, but is more closely associated with anxiety and would more likely respond to a minor tranquilizer than to either type of antidepressant. Difficulty falling asleep *by itself* is not considered a major biological sign of depression. This is important, since the majority of outpatients have neurotic/characterologic or reactive depressions. The latter, generally subside by themselves in three to six months. A history of depressions during some part of the day or lasting two days with a subsequent return to *normal* mood should infer neurotic depression not manic-depressive (bipolar) or unipolar depressions both of which generally last until they are treated with drugs (6 months to 20 years), although they sometimes revert by them-selves, only to recur sometime later. (There are, however, a few manic-depressives who cycle from severe mania to severe depression within 48 hours.)

In general, *unipolar* depressions, characterized by sleep loss (particularly early morning awakening, two hours or more early) plus agitation or severe anxiety and/or somatic complaints, com-bined with loss of appetite and/or weight loss, respond well to *tri-cyclics*.

The tricyclics are:

Elavil (amitriptyline)   Norpramin (desipramine)
                           Aventyl (nortriptyline)
                           Pertofrane (desipramine)
Tofranil (imipramine)   Vivactil (protriptyline)
                           Sinequan (doxepin)

THE absolutely CARDINAL thing to remember about tricyclic antidepressants, and MAOIs is that *response may just BEGIN in two WEEKS or MORE* from the date of starting the treatment. It is crucial that the patient, who is hoping for an instantaneous cure from his depression, be so informed. I generally tell the patient that we will start at a low dose and keep going up at two week intervals until a definite response or no response is apparent.

Please note that many doctors *do not* know the correct dosage of these drugs and tend to underdose, thereby giving the ultimate impression that the tricyclic trial has failed. The *minimum effective* dose for persons under approximately 65 years of age is 100 mg per day of amitriptyline (Elavil) or imipramine (Tofranil) or the equivalent of the other drugs; exceptions are extremely rare. Combination products which combine small doses of phenothiazines with small doses of tricyclics generally do not contain enough tricyclic to get a good antidepressant response if oversedation with the phenothiazine part is to be avoided. For elderly persons with agitated unipolar depressions, however, these drugs may be quite beneficial since elderly persons often respond to lower doses of tricyclics. At any rate, I usually begin treatment at 100 mg. Imipramine or amitriptyline or the equivalent of the other drugs (doxepin 100 mg, desipramine 100 mg, nortriptyline 50 mg, protriptyline 10 mg) for five days to accustom the patient to the few and mild side effects he may experience. The dose is then raised to 150 mg of amitriptyline or imipramine or equivalents of the others, and await the completion of the two weeks. If there is absolutely no improvement in the two weeks, I prescribe 200 mg and wait another two weeks and so on up to 300 mg per day. Again, the dose is not simply dependent on body weight or depth of depression, but is a complex interaction of intestinal absorption, blood level maintenance, blood-brain barrier interactions, and many other factors, the majority of which are still unknown. If after the patient reaches 300 mg for two weeks and there is no response, I will wait an additional week or two before considering the drug a failure. Incidentally, if one tricyclic fails, the others will be *no more* likely to succeed*—unlike the side effect situation with phenothiazines. It is then MEDICALLY and ETHICALLY IMPERATIVE (in the United States) to wait at *least two weeks more* before MAOIs are attempted after discontinuing the tricyclics. (In England MAOIs and tricyclics are sometimes used concomitantly. A few deaths are thought to have resulted

---

*This statement may have to be modified soon since there is now a trickle of research evidence suggesting that there is differential response in the population, some persons only improving on either one or the other of amitriptyline or imipramine.

from the combination and this has led to the combination being specifically contraindicated in the United States.)

This may seem a bit arduous and "trial and error," which it is, but meanwhile the patient is undergoing psychotherapy which hopefully sustains him until the drug begins to work. If the diagnosis is correct and the optimum dose is reached, the response, in a few weeks time, is amazing. Incidentally, in all fairness to everybody's professional ego, such results are more doubtfully obtainable with an equally short term of psychotherapy. (One can never account, however, for "placebo reactions," spontaneous remissions, and so called "transference cures.")

It is also important to keep suicide in mind during the period of deep depression, before the tricyclic begins to work and *ESPECIALLY during the first two weeks after a small response has been noted.* The patient may still be depressed enough to want to kill himself and now as he is emerging from the depression, has the "energy" to do it.

A word about bipolar depressions and tricyclics. The bipolar depression, as you may recall, is characterized generally by excessive sleeping (hypersomnia), weight gain, severe energylessness (anergia), with a *HISTORY* of a hypomanic or manic episodes at any time in the past. If the depression is so characterized but no hypomanic or manic episodes have yet occurred, the patient must be classified as unipolar, although there is a likelihood that at some time such an episode *will* occur in the future. However, it is generally accepted to start even bipolar depressives on tricyclics first (unless it is known that they previously have *not* responded to up to 300 mg) due to the greater *potential* toxicity of the MAOIs. If the bipolar depression does not respond within four weeks after initiating therapy, with more rapid rises in dosage to 300 mg per day, I usually discontinue the tricyclics, *wait two weeks* and initiate treatment with MAO inhibitors. MAO inhibitors are:

Nardil (phenelzine)	Parnate (tranylcypromine)
Actomol (mebanazine)	Marplan (isocarboxazid)
Niamide (nialamide)	Eutonyl (pargyline)

These, like the tricyclics, are all essentially equal and one is not likely to succeed if another has failed. (I have, however, encountered patients who claim a better response to one MAOI than another. Again, this may be due to specific patient-physiology-drug interactions.) There are also arguments that MAO inhibitors can be ranked from weakest to strongest as follows. Marplan, Nardil, Eutonyl, Niamide, Parnate, Actomol. This presumably refers to milligram for milligram potency in inhibiting MAO enzyme. However, once the weak MAOI is given in an appropriately high dosage, it should be equal in effect to the more potent MAOI's. However, this in itself needs modification, since MAO enzyme has several forms which may be differentially inhibited by the various MAOI's. In fact there is recent evidence that, because of the differential inhibition, e.g. the brain MAO enzyme vs. the peripheral enzyme, some people can get an antidepressant effect yet can eat the MAOI diet-prohibited foods without ill-effect. All this is to say that the state of this science is such, that we do not know enough to know who will respond to which drug, and that, therefore, although it is unlikely to succeed, it is still worth a try to change from one MAOI to a stronger one, provided that you have waited two weeks in between.

The problem with MAO inhibitors is that the patient must be *extremely reliable.* I mean that he has to follow certain food restrictions or risk the possibility of severe blood pressure increase, which has occasionally caused some deaths or strokes. Bipolar patients may also become hypomanic or manic during treatment with MAOIs, may lose judgment and eat or drink forbidden items. If the patient tends to get too "high" from MAOIs (or tricyclics for that matter), lithium is the treatment of choice, in combination with antidepressants. As you can see, the treatment of manic-depressive illness might initially be better carried out by a psychiatrist or internist familiar with these drugs. Once regulated on lithium with or without antidepressants, psychotherapy can proceed, if warranted, now that the patient's mood swings are regulated. Lithium serum levels after initial regulation should be done at least once a month and should generally be kept at 0.9 mEq/liter to 1.2 mEq/liter; however, some patients respond at both lower and higher serum levels. With lithium (as well as MAOIs) the patient must be extremely reliable since the toxic dose of lithium is exceedingly close to the therapeutic dose and may differ only by one capsule of lithium carbonate. At any rate, except for the dietary restrictions, MAOIs are practically free of side effects and are very valuable for bipolar and some unipolar depressions, with or without psychosis. They may be the only antidepressants that work for certain people and they are invaluable because of this.

The dietary restrictions are as follows:

NO *cheese, red wine, beer,* pickled herring, sour cream, yogurt, chicken livers, canned figs, raisins, CHOCOLATE, soy sauce, fava beans or lima beans. Cottage cheese is okay.

There are restrictions *also* on types of medicine NOT to be taken with MAO inhibitors under *any* circumstances.

NO cold tablets or cold medicines of *any* type (no nose spray either). *NO* amphetamines, diet pills, mood elevators, etc. *NO TRICYCLICS* (In the United States). NO L-DOPA. *NO* antihistamines of certain types (The PDR should be referenced).

Obviously, the patient has to be willing to carry around his list of forbidden foods and drugs. I personally have treated numerous patients as outpatients who were taking MAO inhibitors. I generally tell them that attempting suicide with restricted foods or drugs will generally not result in death (which is true) but may result in severe headache, nosebleeds or stroke, with paralysis possibly leaving them *helplessly* alive. I also give them a great deal of moral support about needing to wait two weeks before the antidepressant effects start, and I see them two or three times a week during this period (as I do with any suicidal patient). Again, the most crucial time is when the patient is just beginning to emerge from the depression. A special problem is the formerly anergic patient, who now feels energetic enough to commit suicide and is still depressed enough to want to.

You may begin to think that MAO inhibitors are drastic measures. Certainly in many respects, tricyclics are potentially safer. But depression, either unipolar or bipolar is a potentially *lethal* disease and somewhat risky measures need to be employed to combat it. With a patient who knows he has your support you can safely give either tricyclics or MAOIs provided the risk of suicide is not so great that the patient ought to be hospitalized. The dose is very variable and depends on which drug is used.

Side Effects

The main side effect of both tricyclics and MAOIs is orthostatic hypotension, the same as occurs in phenothiazines. You may remember that orthostatic hypotension is temporarily low blood pressure with change in position from lying down or sitting to standing. Tricyclics also have a high incidence of anticholinergic side effects like dry mouth, stuffy nose, constipation, difficulty in urination, palpitations, etc. They do not generally have "Parkinsonian" side effects although chemically they resemble phenothiazines very closely. Tricyclics have been used, sucessfully, in combating enuresis (bed wetting) in young boys. They are also used successfully sometimes in severe chronic pain although the mechanism (aside from the depressing element of chronic pain) is unknown. Tricyclics may cause sedation (amitriptyline (Elavil) and doxepin (Sinequan) being the more sedative, but the others having similar potential) which may be a rather beneficial side effect in persons with difficulty falling asleep as well as early morning awakening. Tricyclics may also cause blurring of near vision as with phenothiazines. On the other hand, MAOIs, with the exception of diet and drug restrictions and orthostatic hypotension are virtually free of side effects. They may cause dry mouth or palpitations, but these are less frequent than with tricyclics. One point to note about tranylcypromine (Parnate) in particular is that, possibly because of its resemblance to amphetamine, it can cause difficulty in getting to sleep if taken close to bedtime. I have had patients who complained of difficulty falling asleep with other MAOIs as well. Sometimes taking the total dose before 3 P.M. has been helpful. Since the action of MAOIs does not depend upon maintaining a constant blood level of the drug it can be taken in divided doses, all before 3 P.M. in the afternoon.

LITHIUM

Lithium carbonate (the form used in the United States) is not always an antidepressant by itself. When it is, however, it is generally effective for bipolar patients. There is growing evidence that it *protects* bipolar patients from recurrent attacks of depression while not always really being able to alleviate the depression once it exists. There is newer evidence that lithium also prevents recurrent depression in those people so inclined even though they have never had a manic or hypomanic episode. Sometimes it can prevent recurrent attacks of depression alone, other times MAOIs or tricyclics are used in combination with it. It is certainly well established as an antimanic drug, and protects the patient from excessively high moods where he may do or say socially inappropriate things.

In the future, lithium will come into greater use than it currently has, since there is also growing evidence that it protects persons so inclined from excessively violent or hostile behavior. It is an excellent drug with one exception and that is, *that the effective dose is very close to the toxic dose.* This means that very quickly after reaching therapeutic blood levels, the patient can become physically ill from it if the blood level goes too high. Lithium treatment is best carried out by a psychiatrist at first, until a stable dosage is reached. It has very few, if any, side effects, unless and until the patient becomes "toxic." The first signs of this are nausea and vomiting and gross hand tremors. A hand tremor *alone*, very fine type of tremor is usually present when therapeutic levels are obtained and you can reassure the patient on this point.

The combination of lithium and MAOIs is becoming quite well recognized as the treatment of choice for bipolar illness. There is small, but growing evidence that lithium might prevent recurrent attacks of unipolar depression as well.

CANDIDACY FOR LITHIUM

There is a tremendous amount of publicity being given to lithium by some very prominent people who have been helped by it. This causes a lot of patients to ask psychotherapists and other mental health professionals whether lithium would be of benefit in their case. Some even come in demanding lithium. Most of the patients who want lithium are depressed, and they think they have heard that lithium works in depression. All the evidence is not in yet, and that which is, is equivocal on whether or not lithium is a good antidepressant, even in bipolar depressions. In general, if a person has had *recurrent* CLINICALLY SIGNIFICANT depressions, with or without a history of mania, they should be considered for treatment with lithium. Certainly if they are presently significantly hypomanic or manic with attendant sleep loss, appetite change, weight loss, excess motor activity, etc., they are a prime candidate for lithium. In addition to these more clear-cut indications the situations in which Lithium is used or might be used are various and multiple.

Most of the time a person who has had one single episode of depression wants to know if he needs lithium. This really depends upon the psychiatrist who would prescribe the lithium. In a case like this, however, it would indeed be spurious to say that lithium prevented a recurrence of the depression, if we do not know if it would have recurred if *no* treatment were given. I therefore first treat the depression with either tricyclics or MAOIs. Once the depression has responded, I withdraw the antidepressant after a variable period of time. If the depression recurs within 3 years I use antidepressants again, but would then consider the person for lithium. It is then obvious that there is relapse without some continuous intervention, which then justifies treatment with a potentially toxic drug like lithium.

CHAPTER X

Sedatives, Hypnotics, and Narcotic Analgesics

All the drugs discussed in this chapter are addictive and widely abused by both older and younger generations. It was mentioned that the minor tranquilizers are also addictive, in high doses.

Addiction is a complex interaction of *psychological* and *physical dependence* on a drug. Physical dependence denotes an altered state of the physiology of the person such that stopping the drug will result in a characteristic withdrawal or abstinence syndrome. Most withdrawal syndromes have psychological characteristics, but in order for a drug to truly be considered addictive it must be able to produce *physical* symptoms of withdrawal, usually having a characteristic pattern for that class of drugs. Other components of addiction as defined by the World Health Organization are: 1) an overwhelming desire or need (compulsion) to continue taking the drug and to *obtain it by any means*; 2) a tendency to increase the dose; 3) a detrimental effect on the individual and on society.

The tendency to increase the dose is due to the phenomenon of tolerance; that is, the original dose of the drug no longer produces the original effect, it produces a decreasing effect, so increasingly more of the drug has to be taken to obtain the original response. In general, if a person is tolerant to one specific drug, say Seconal (a barbiturate) he will be tolerant to all barbiturates, and may also be tolerant to other drugs which produce the *same effects* even though they are chemically different. Another point of interest is that drugs that produce the *same effects* (even though chemically dissimilar) will produce very similar withdrawal symptoms.

One very important point to remember is that *withdrawal syndromes generally produce symptoms which are the direct opposite of the usual effects of the drug.* For example, barbiturates generally depress nervous excitability, so you can expect that the withdrawal from barbiturates will cause increased excitability, nervousness, and irritability. This will be clearer when each class of drugs has been discussed.

SEDATIVES AND HYPNOTICS, TYPE I: BARBITURATES

A sedative is a drug that is supposed to decrease excitement and anxiety without producing marked drowsiness. Hypnotic, for our purposes, is really a misnomer and actually should be called soporific or simply sleep-producing. Barbiturates are medically used as both sedatives and sleeping pills. Whether they act as a sedative or produce sleep depends on the dose. Unfortunately even in small doses most patients complain of drowsiness when a barbiturate is prescribed to calm anxiety.

Barbiturates are much abused in today's society. They are used to get intoxicated ("high") and they are used for sleep by many, as part of what I call the "up and down" syndrome—amphetamines during the day ("ups" as they are called) and barbiturates at night ("downs") because the person can't sleep at night due to the "ups" he took during the day and can't wake up in the morning due to the "downs" he took the night before.

Here is a list of the trade and "street" names of the most commonly prescribed and, for that matter, abused, barbiturates. Their most common medical use is also listed. Many other preparations, not used exclusively as sedatives or sleeping pills, contain barbiturates, but that list is too long to be included. Barbiturates in general are called downs, goofballs, barbs, and idiot pills.

Brand Name	Medical Use	Street Names
Butisol (butabarbital)	sedative and sleep	
Luminal (phenobarbital)	sedative and sleep	
Amytal (amobarbital)	sedative and sleep	
Seconal (secobarbital)	sleep	red devils, red birds, red 88's, reds
Nembutal (pentobarbital)	sleep	yellow jackets, nemmies
Tuinal (secobarbital plus amobarbital)	sleep	rainbows, tooies, double trouble

The Effects of Barbiturates

At the most basic level, barbiturates interfere with certain groups of cells in the brain which are responsible for alertness. A barbiturate is one type of central nervous system depressant; that is, it tends to depress (slow down, decrease) many functions of the brain and spinal cord (which, taken together, are called the central nervous system). As far as we are concerned here, barbiturates slow down speech, respiration, body movements, thinking, and the capacity to verbalize thoughts. People intoxicated ("stoned") on barbiturates look very much the same as though they were drunk on alcohol. Their balance is impaired, they may stagger or drag their feet, their eyes look sort of half-open or drowsy, and their movements may be uncoordinated. However, many addicts can take barbiturates all day long and although they are psychologically "high," they somehow manage not to show most of the signs of intoxication except if you are very alert to a slight slurring of speech and a slight slowing of their ability to verbalize thoughts.

An overdose of barbiturates can produce anything from

prolonged sleep to death by respiratory arrest (the center in the brain controlling automatic breathing simply stops; the person, already sleeping or in a coma, stops breathing). A good rule of thumb, for patients who need sleeping pills and are suicidal, is that one weeks supply (usually seven pills) is unlikely to cause death even if taken at once. However, the effects of alcohol, tranquilizers, narcotics, and nonbarbiturate sleeping pills are additive to the effect of barbiturates. Therefore, keep these additive effects in mind when assessing the suicidal potential of a given prescription.

The person addicted to barbiturates of any type is tolerant to them and tends to take as many as he can get his hands on. He will also consume nonbarbiturate sleeping pills since they have the same effect and, hence, he is tolerant to them also (crosstolerance).

The clinical description of barbiturate intoxication has already been presented. It should be noted that it is very similar to alcohol intoxication, and that like alcoholics, barbiturate addicts can hide most of the clinical effects from you.

A Further Note On Effects

Unlike the effects of chronic alcohol intoxication, which can be permanent brain and liver damage, and a host of other permanent damages, chronic barbiturate intoxication *of itself* is not to my knowledge associated with any *permanent* damage to any organ or to the brain. No matter how long the patient has been addicted or chronically intoxicated, once he is withdrawn safely, there do not seem to be permanent ill effects. The problem is that like heroin and alcohol addiction, the life style and eating habits of the barbiturate addict deteriorate. There is general body neglect and often disease if the addict injects the drugs by vein. Also, many addicts suffer from vitamin deficiencies and very poor dental hygiene.

Permanent brain damage can result, however, from overdosage, with ensuing coma and inadequate supply of oxygen caused by too shallow breathing for too long. Brain damage can also result from uncontrolled convulsions which can result from barbiturate withdrawal.

If your patient admits to barbiturate addiction, or if you suspect he is addicted, you must remember one absolutely unbreakable rule: NEVER, UNDER ANY CIRCUMSTANCES TELL A BARBITURATE ADDICT TO STOP TAKING BARBITURATES ABRUPTLY. ABRUPT WITHDRAWAL OF BARBITURATES CAN RESULT IN UNCONTROLLABLE CONVULSIONS AND DEATH. A barbiturate addict cannot go "cold turkey." If he wants to withdraw, he should be kept in a hospital where access to supply is limited and where he can be gradually withdrawn safely.

You may come across a patient addict who does not know the above fact, and may have decided to stop taking his barbiturates abruptly. If the withdrawal syndrome has already begun, he will be irritable, hypersensitive to environmental stimuli (e.g., noise), highly anxious, tremulous, and may complain of nausea and abdominal pain. If he is further into withdrawal he may present signs of delirium, i.e., confusion, memory impairment, disorientation, as well as hyperirritability. In any case, as a stop-gap measure, tell him to take one or two barbiturates immediately, and then get him to a hospital right away—because all of these signs precede convulsions.

A Rough Guide To Tell If Your Patient Is Addicted

A person can be mildly physically dependent on as few as two Nembutal, Seconal or Tuinal per day, in that he might experience hyperexcitability and nervousness if he suddenly stops taking them. If he is only taking two per day every day, he is *unlikely* to experience convulsions upon withdrawal. If a patient is taking only one or two barbiturates a day and *doesn't* tend to increase the dose, but wants to continue them for sleep and does *not* get withdrawal symptoms if he doesn't take them, he is said to be *habituated*. Habituation involves *psychological* but not *physical dependence*.

In my own practice I would even hesitate to tell a patient who I felt I was absolutely *sure* was taking *only* two barbiturates a day to stop taking them, because the likelihood is that if a patient is admitting to two a day, he is taking more like four a day or more, so it is advisable to get him into a drug detoxification unit at a hospital if he wants to withdraw.

There is no upper limit to the number of pills per day that defines addiction, but four Seconal, Nembutal or Tuinal per day can produce a clinically significant physical dependence.

In true addiction, the tendency is to increase the dose of one specific drug, or take other drugs whose effects are the same in combination—whatever the addict can get his hands on. In trying to assess a patient's drug intake be sure to ask about nonbarbiturate sleeping pills and minor tranquilizers, etc.

There are no real *clinical* signs of barbiturate *addiction* per se, if the drugs are not injected, but there are those signs of intoxication and withdrawal which we have mentioned. If a patient suddenly complains of anxiety, irritability and hypersensitivity to noise, light etc. ask him if he had been taking barbiturates and stopped, even if he never admitted it to you before. You may save his life.

SEDATIVES AND HYPNOTICS, TYPE II: NONBARBITURATE PRESCRIPTION DRUGS

The drugs covered in this section are generally medically used for sleep rather than as antianxiety sedatives. They all have additive effects with alcohol, tranquilizers, barbiturates, and narcotics. Some are chemically very similar to barbiturates, others are very different, but all have the capacity to induce sleep or intoxication in chronic abusers and all are addictive. In general, addicts tolerant to barbiturates will be tolerant to these drugs too, and vice versa. Most do not, in themselves, produce any permanent organ or brain damage, even after years of chronic ingestion or intoxication. The withdrawal symptoms in general are very similar to those produced by discontinuance of barbiturates and the same warning is given here as is given for those drugs: NEVER TELL A SLEEPING-PILL ADDICT TO ABRUPTLY STOP TAKING SLEEPING PILLS AS THIS CAN RESULT IN UNCONTROLLABLE CONVULSIONS AND DEATH.

In general, the results of overdosage with nonbarbiturate sleeping pills are the same as those with barbiturates, namely anything from prolonged sleep to coma and death by respiratory arrest.

You may have been wondering why there are different types of barbiturates and why, if the effects are so similar, the nonbarbiturate sleeping pills were developed at all. Free enterprise is one answer, but also the drugs do vary in their speed of onset of action, how long they keep the person asleep, and how fast they are eliminated by the body. Some of these variables determine, for example, how much of a "hangover" a given drug produces the following day. Also, there is always the problem of allergy to barbiturates and individual drug sensitivities, tolerance, or preferences.

The most commonly prescribed drugs in this category of nonbarbiturate sleeping preparations are:

Chloral hydrate	(This is the generic name)
Paraldehyde	(This is the generic name)
Placidyl	(ethchlorvynol)
Valmid	(ethinamate)
Doriden	(glutethimide)
Noludar	(methyprylon)
Dalmane	(flurazepam)
Quaalude	(methaqualone)

NARCOTIC-ANALGESICS: OPIUM DERIVATIVES AND SYNTHETIC NARCOTICS

Opium is derived from the unripe seed capsules of the opium poppy (*Papaver somniferum*). Two of the natural products of opium have narcotic (producing numbness and/or lethargy) analgesic (pain relieving) effects. These are morphine and codeine. Heroin is produced synthetically from morphine and is also a very potent narcotic-analgesic. In fact, heroin was once introduced as a cure for addiction to morphine, having all of its pain-relieving qualities, but allegedly none of its addicting properties. Unfortunately, this was not so, and science is still searching for the potent analgesic that is nonaddicting. All of the drugs in the following list are addictive. Many are synthetically derived from morphine or codeine and others are entirely synthetically produced. All of the drugs are cross tolerant with each other—every single one of them. An addict can take any one of them for at least partial relief from withdrawal symptoms due to another. The list is long and may contain a surprise or two, like Darvon (Darvon is weakly addictive), but it will serve as a reference, in case one of your patients has had one of them prescribed, became mildly addicted, and begins to experience withdrawal symptoms.

Dilaudid	(hydromorphone)
Percodan	(oxycodone is the narcotic, but Percodan also contains aspirin, phenacetin and caffeine)
Demerol	(meperidine)
Dolophine	(methadone) (Prescription limited in U.S.)
Darvon	(Propoxyphene)
Codeine	generic
Morphine	generic
Heroin	(cannot be prescribed (generic) in U.S.)

There are many others, but these are the most common.

The Effects Of Narcotic-Analgesics

All of the drugs on the above list are powerful pain relievers, but some are much less potent than others in the usually prescribed dose. Depending upon the circumstances they relieve anxiety and fear as well. Morphine and heroin and to a lesser extent all the others are said by addicts to produce euphoria, but many persons respond negatively to the feeling-state produced by these drugs. They also very frequently cause drowsiness, dizziness, and nausea. All produce constipation and to some extent may cause difficulty in urinating and/or a decrease in urine volume. All are powerful respiratory depressants, and death from overdosage is almost always due to respiratory arrest. Morphine and heroin and to a lesser extent the rest of the drugs markedly decrease sexual desire and may also delay ejaculation or inhibit it completely. An important clinical note is that heroin and morphine, as well as some of the others, produce very marked constriction of the pupils; a telltale sign of whether a patient has had a dose within the last four hours. (One exception is Demerol which produces dilation (widening) of the pupils.)

It is again interesting that chronic abuse of these drugs does *not* cause permanent damage to any organ or the brain in and of itself. However, because many addicts inject the drugs into their veins, hepatitis (liver infection) and infection of the lining of the heart (bacterial endocarditis) often occur due to the lack of sterile conditions during injection, and can result in permanent damage to these organs. Continuous injection in the same vein—even with a sterile needle—can result in inflammation and clotting of the blood in the vein.

There are no definite always present outward signs of addiction per se, but certain points are worth mentioning. Needle tracks on the arms or legs may be present. These are often long, reddened or darker-colored streaks which follow the course of veins, on the skin of the forearm or inside portion of the ankles and calves. Many addicts *always* wear long sleeved shirts, even in summer, to hide these tracks, plus wearing sunglasses indoors to hide constriction of the pupils. These signs should alert you but many addicts inject under the skin ("skin-popping") and do not have needle tracks. However, "skin-poppers" often have many boils and small infections on their arms. An addict who has just injected heroin may have slurred speech, incoordination and slow thinking or verbalization, just as a barbiturate addict or alcoholic may have. But I have seen hundreds of addicts who, if it were not for needle tracks or constricted pupils, show no other outward signs of having just injected.

The Abstinence (Withdrawal) Syndrome Characteristic For Drugs Listed

Heroin will be used as a model, but these symptoms occur upon withdrawal of any of the drugs listed, if the patient is addicted.

The symptoms usually begin in 6-12 hours after the last dose. They are: yawning, eyes tearing, nose dripping clear fluid, and sweating. Later on, over the next 12-24 hours, the patient gets muscle cramps and muscle twitches, hot and cold flashes, chills and dilation of the pupils.* (Since many of the early signs are subjective and can be faked I never believe an addict who complains he is in withdrawal unless his pupils are dilated.) About 36-48 hours after the last dose, the patient will vomit, wretch, have diarrhea, refuse to eat or drink very much, and will continue to twitch and complain of pain in his back and legs. On about the third day after the last dose most of these symptoms will have subsided, but the patient may continue to complain of weakness, back and leg pain or cramps, insomnia and restlessness for days to weeks after withdrawal.

As you can see, this withdrawal syndrome is not nearly as dangerous as the convulsions that ensue from sleeping-pill withdrawal and many addicts have gone through it without medical aid ("cold turkey"). It *is* more humane, however, to have the patient admitted to a drug detoxification center than to let him go "cold turkey."

Methadone

Methadone and methadone maintenance are the subjects of considerable controversy. Methadone is pharmacologically similar to morphine and heroin in that it is addictive and it alleviates pain. It is much longer acting than morphine and is said not to produce the same "high" as heroin. Methadone has also been said to be capable of "blocking" the "high" from heroin if taken before it. Methadone is cross tolerant with all the drugs listed and can be used as a substitute for them to lessen withdrawal symptoms. The one advantage of methadone is that it can be taken orally but, aside from heroin and morphine, so can all the other drugs listed. It is interesting to think about why society and the medical community sanction methadone for maintenance as opposed to any other of the oral drugs, or why, if it is so similar to heroin and as addictive, we don't have heroin maintenance. There really are many arguments pro and con about methadone and heroin maintenance, but these are quite beyond the scope of this book.

*Demerol is the exception, constriction occurs when this drug is used.

Maintenance means just what it says: the addict is placed on high doses of methadone initially to substitute for his heroin habit and gradually the dosage is decreased but not discontinued, and the addict then comes to a methadone maintenance center for his daily dose. Many addicts feel that methadone prevents their craving for heroin, and since it is legal and free, they do not have to engage in illegal activities to obtain either the heroin or money to get it.

CHAPTER XI

Psychotomimetics

The drugs discussed in this chapter are all capable of producing hallucinations; one of the hallmarks of psychosis. However, they can produce profound alterations in thinking and mood as well, which can be indistinguishable from psychotic states—hence they are called psychotomimetic rather than merely hallucinogenic.

Psychotomimetic drugs produce sensory illusions (distortions of perception based on some object or occurrence in reality), hallucinations (sensory perceptions generated entirely by the mind), distortions of time sense and body image, increased vividness of perception, memory or fantasy, and depersonalization (the subject feels strangely detached from himself and may feel like he is watching himself going through the experience). Changes in mood generally go in the direction of euphoria, but on "bad trips" there can be profound depression or panic. Delusions occur also and can be mild (flashes of great "insight" which later turn out to be gibberish) or severe (wherein the person feels people are out to kill him or that he is going to die, etc). Protracted psychotic reactions do occur with these drugs and these are, or are sometimes indistinguishable from, acute schizophrenic states. There is some evidence that schizophrenic reactions following these drugs are not really caused by them, but merely released by the drugs. (A protracted reaction is usually considered to be one where the person is still either hallucinating, delusional, panicked or depressed, etc., three days after drug ingestion.)

With the exception of amphetamines, none of the psychotomimetics cause physical dependence, nor do they have abstinence syndrome. Prolonged and high-dose use of these drugs can lead to personality changes which are slowly becoming recognized as "loss of motivation" syndromes.

LSD, MESCALINE, DMT, STP (DOM), PSILOCYBIN, NUTMEG, DOET

These drugs grouped taken together because they are essentially similar in effects. (STP and DOET are really amphetamine derivatives, but are more closely allied to the others than to prescribable amphetamines as they will be discussed later in this chapter.) It is important to realize that psychosis *is* the *usual* (and usually desired) effect of these drugs, produced by *one* sufficient dose of the drug. This is in contrast to amphetamines and marijuana which *are* psychotomimetic, but psychosis is *not* the *usual* or expected response, with one dose.

The drugs are generally taken orally and rarely (except STP) if ever injected. They take effect usually within one hour if an ample dose is taken. At first there are some sympathetic effects—pupil dilatation, increased heart rate, and increased blood pressure. Soon the psychotomimetic effects begin and the subject usually feels euphoric and may begin to have visual illusions like walls undulating or his feet going further away from him. He then may begin to hallucinate. It is interesting that with psychotomimetics, unlike psychosis itself, the subject usually retains the insight that the experiences he is undergoing are unreal. Occasionally the person on LSD, STP or the other drugs for that matter, may show signs of acute organic brain syndrome with its disorientation and memory impairment. In that case the state would be called a toxic psychosis. Usually, however, the subject knows where he is and what day it is, but is too distracted by his hallucinations or his euphoria, to tell you.

Flashbacks can occur with any of these drugs. These are the occurrence of illusions, delusions, hallucinations or any other components of the psychedelic experience, days, weeks or months *after* the *last ingestion.* I had a patient who had taken amphetamines and LSD rather steadily for a month, and was still complaining of walls undulating, wallpaper patterns "flowing" and depersonalization two years after his last ingestion. In this case, as in many others, it is likely that his psychopathology was released by the drug rather than caused by it.

There is no treatment necessary for the ingestion of these drugs, unless the person is panicked or is on a "bad trip" and wants relief. Overdose is rare, but can warrant medical attention mostly for the psychological ill effects. If you have a patient who is having a "bad trip," the best thing to do is get him to the emergency room of a hospital. There he will be treated with phenothiazines or benzodiazepines to which most of the drug-effects respond. The treatment of a patient who has had a schizophrenic reaction following LSD or other drug ingestion, is generally the same as if it were not apparently initiated by the drug experience. The patient is treated with phenothiazines and the appropriate psychotherapy.

Long Range Effects

Certainly, all the evidence is not in yet, and the evidence which *is* in is contradictory. Some studies have shown increases in chromosomal breakage in LSD users. Other studies found no difference in frequency of such breakage between users and nonusers. Memory defects have been found by some investigators, and are disputed by others. I have personally had patients who *complain* of memory defects years after heavy LSD use, but these defects are very difficult to demonstrate on objective testing.

While subtle changes in memory and other intellectual functions may be difficult to document, psychological changes have been well documented. At the present time there is no doubt that the most serious *known* possible consequence of psychotomimetic drug use (whether one dose or heavy use) is protracted psychotic disturbance, markedly resembling schizophrenia. It is difficult to know in such cases whether the "schizophrenia" is a drug effect, or a latent process which has been uncovered or released by the drug. Some studies show that protracted reactions occur usually after high doses or prolonged usage in persons who have a history of previous psychological or neurological disturbance. However, even this is disputed, and other studies indicate that prolonged psychotic reactions occur in persons with no previous psychiatric history.

Most of the studies have been done on LSD users. This does not detract from the psychotogenic potential of the other drugs, but in a way, may even enhance it. This is because few LSD users use only LSD, and often combine it with mescaline, amphetamines or STP. It therefore becomes difficult to know which drug has caused the protracted psychosis. It is safe to say that *any* psychotomimetic is capable of producing or uncovering a schizophrenic-like syndrome which may last for weeks to months or even years after ingestion.

AMPHETAMINES AND AMPHETAMINE-COGENERS

Trade Names Amphetamines	Specific	"Street" Name	General Names
Benzedrine Dexedrine Bontril	(amphetamine sulfate)	bennies	"ups," pep pills
Amodex Obotan Bamadex	(dextroamphetamine)	dexies	speed, diet pills
Desbutal Desoxyn Fetamin Obedrine	(methamphetamine)	meth, crystal	
Biphetamine	(amphetamine and destroamphetamine)	black beauties	cross countries
Amphetamine cogeners			
Ritalin Preludin	(methyphenidate) (phenmetrazine)		

Amphetamines are very widely used and abused by all segments of the population, from college student to doctors and nurses, to dieters everywhere. All the drugs on the above list are legal by prescription in the United States, but are presently *controlled drugs*, much like morphine or barbiturates. The *more* psychotogenic amphetamine derivatives (STP, DOET) are not legally prescribable. However, amphetamines and cogeners of the type discussed in this section *are definitely psychotomimetic.* The difference is that the prescribable amphetamines and cogeners do *not regularly* and *usually* produce hallucinations, illusions, etc. with *one* dose. In order to obtain psychotic reactions from these, high and frequent doses must be taken. These amphetamines, however, are *addicting.* They produce a withdrawal syndrome whose symptoms are indicative of psychological and physical dependence. As with any addictive drug, tolerance develops, so the user must increase his dose in order to get the same effect.

Amphetamines are central nervous system stimulants, and their effects physiologically closely parallel sympathetic stimulation. That is, they cause nervousness, irritability, loss of appetite, insomnia, increased blood pressure, increased heart rate, sweating, and pupil dilatation. It is from some of these properties that the amphetamines derive their medical uses. They are often prescribed for weight reduction because of their ability to suppress appetite. The appetite-suppression effect is very short-lived, however, so that amphetamines can only be taken effectively for dieting for about two weeks. Amphetamines are also prescribed to help keep people awake who suffer from a type of epilepsy in which the patient gets attacks of sleep (narcolepsy). Most unfortunately, amphetamines or cogeners are frequently prescribed for temporary relief of depression. Here again their effect lasts only about two weeks. If no more long-lasting antidepressant is prescribed during the course of the amphetamines, the person may feel as bad or worse at the end of those two weeks due to the let down secondary to the reduced effectiveness of the amphetamines as when he began.

Psychologically, amphetamines produce euphoria, increased sexual drive, excitement, "high," or fearfulness, ideas of reference, paranoid feelings, hallucinations, delusions, and violent impulsive behavior, depending upon the dose, frequency of the dose and whether the use is one dose or chronic. In an experiment, "normal" volunteers were given amphetamines intravenously (by vein) until psychosis was reached. All the subjects experienced a paranoid psychosis almost indistinguishable from paranoid schizophrenia within two to five days of continuous hourly infusion. Before becoming psychotic, however, all the subjects went through a period of depression and social withdrawal, even though they were still receiving the amphetamine.

Chronic abuse of amphetamines in high doses can interfere with mental functioning and motivation for several years after withdrawal. As with any addiction, deterioration in health and social functioning occurs, and this is worsened by the poor appetite and insomnia caused by the drug. The danger of inducing a paranoid schizophrenia-like syndrome remains ever present if amphetamines are used in high doses over time.

It is very interesting that the above statements apply only to *adults*. Amphetamines or cogeners are prescribed in frequent doses to very young children who are "hyperactive" presumably as a result of minimal brain damage. In children, amphetamines act to increase attention span and ability to concentrate, this combination tends to make the child appear less hyperactive and distractable. Children treated with relatively high doses (for them) do not usually become psychotic even with treatment over long periods of time.

Amphetamine Withdrawal

Although the full physiological and psychological withdrawal syndrome occurs only after tolerance and addiction have developed, even one dose or occasional use of amphetamines can result in a post-drug depression or lethargy. This is why these drugs should not be used as antidepressants. The full withdrawal syndrome is a psychological disaster. As if it were not enough that high frequent doses produce a paranoid psychosis during abuse, withdrawal also produces a paranoid psychosis, equally indistinguishable from paranoid schizophrenia. Frightening hallucinations, both auditory and visual occur, and paranoid delusions are common. Extreme lethargy, depression, and fatigue are the rule, since these are the direct opposite effects of the drug. The amphetamine addict who is "crashing" may sleep for several days, but this sleep is disturbed both physiologically and psychologically. Terrifying nightmares occur, and EEG recordings demonstrate severe abnormalities of REM sleep (rapid eye movement stage of sleep) during this period. Headaches, profuse sweating, and severe muscle cramping accompany the psychological symptoms. Even if psychotic symptoms do not occur, withdrawal is marked by severe depression, and terrifying thoughts or feelings.

The amphetamine abstinence psychosis generally begins a few days after discontinuing use, but this reaction has been known to occur as long as two months later. It usually lasts about a week, but again, may persist for months or years and progress to a chronic phase indistinguishable from chronic paranoid schizophrenia.

Obviously, an amphetamine addict who wants to withdraw, should be withdrawn in a hospital, not only because psychosis may possibly occur, but because the depression which accompanies the withdrawal presents a significant suicide risk.

COCAINE

Cocaine is a central nervous system stimulant and resembles the action of amphetamines very closely. It does not, however, produce physical dependence or tolerance. It does produce one of the strongest cravings known in drug abuse. Craving may be an as yet unmeasurable physiological response, but it is certainly a marked psychological response. Cocaine, amphetamines, and heroin are about equal in their ability to produce almost overwhelming desire for themselves long after cessation. This craving is so strong that it usually leads to resumption of abuse, even though cocaine is not physically addicting.

Cocaine produces the familiar sympathetic effects noted for amphetamines, but in addition has the capacity to produce convulsions. It *is* psychotomimetic and large doses can produce delusions, hallucinations, and paranoid ideation.

MARIJUANA AND HASHISH

Marijuana and hashish come from plants of the genus *cannabis*. The active ingredient in both plants is tetrahydrocannabinol or THC. It is THC which produces the psychoactive effects of these two drugs. Hashish has the higher content of THC. THC is found in different quantities in different parts of the plant. In general the THC content is found in decreasing quantity in the following parts: resin, flowers, leaves. There is practically no THC in the stems, roots or seeds. Jamaican ganja is more potent than marijuana because it is made from the flower tops and some leaves. Hashish is made exclusively from the resin and is the most potent of the THC-containing drugs.

Since the psychoactive ingredient is THC, both drugs exert similar effects on the mental functioning of the user. Hashish will produce a greater effect and last longer since it contains more THC than the other products.

The route by which the drugs are taken generally affects the time lapse until drug effect is felt and the duration of the response, but all routes—generally smoking or eating—will ultimately produce a response if sufficient quantity is taken. High doses can be psychotomimetic.

Psychotic phenomena such as hallucinations, mild delusions, distortion of body image, and loss of sense of identity can occur. Also, and not to be confused with psychotic phenomena, panic reactions or anxiety reactions can occur, especially in novice users. These reactions occur when the person is afraid that his sense of subjective self-control is lost, or is terrified that he is losing his mind or sense of identity. Both psychotic phenomena and panic reactions clear rapidly as the THC is eliminated from the body.

Tolerance to THC (by long-term users) is said (by them) to occur, but apparently physical addiction does not. There are claims for both straight tolerance, i.e., more drug needed to produce usual response, and "reverse tolerance", i.e., *less* drug needed the more is consumed on previous occasions. In recent months I have heard arguments for both possibilities. The arguments are usually based on how rapidly different metabolites are excreted or stored. Psychological dependence does occur where the taking of the drug becomes a compulsive necessity in order to "feel good" or even "feel normal." This leads to drug-seeking behavior which is tantamount to the type of drug-seeking behavior found with drugs like heroin which are physically addicting.

The Marijuana Commission Report National Commission, (1972) does not conclusively state that brain injury occurs with extremely heavy use. They do note, however, that pulmonary (lung) function is decreased as with any chronic smoking, but mostly in those who smoke regular cigarettes.

Studies done in other countries where hashish has been smoked heavily for periods of 20 years or more, indicate evidence of motivation changes and other changes in behavior which accommodate the drug-seeking and compulsive behaviors associated with very heavy use.

With *intermittent "social"* use, *no behavioral, physical,* or *mental changes* could be demonstrated. This is also true of alcohol whose deleterious effects of chronic use are more clear-cut than those for long-term heavy THC ingestion. It is interesting that the Commission on Marijuana recommended continued prohibition of marijuana essentially because of the risk of increasing the number of long-term heavy users; despite the fact that the predominant use in this country is short term and intermittent. The Commission concluded that the existing social and legal policies relating to marijuana use were out of proportion to the demonstrable social or physical harm which could come from such use. This is in marked contrast to society's view of alcohol whose deleterious effects on mind and body are very well known, but whose use is unrestricted.

CHAPTER XII

Alcohol and Alcoholism

ALCOHOL AS A DRUG

Alcohol is a central nervous system depressant. As you may recall from other chapters, this means that it slows down the functions of higher and lower brain and spinal cord centers. It is similar therefore to major and minor tranquilizers, barbiturates, narcotics, and nonbarbiturate sleeping pills. It is additive to the effects of any of these other drugs. It is psychologically and physically addictive in that there is a specific withdrawal syndrome that occurs if the addicted person stops drinking suddenly. Overdoses *usually* produce sleep before the person can drink enough to suppress his respirations enough to cause death, but overdose can produce death by respiratory arrest. Also, death by respiratory arrest can and often does occur when alcohol is combined with other CNS depressants either by accident or design. In small doses, alcohol is a minor tranquilizer in that it produces emotional relaxation for a short period of time. It is also a vasodilator, that is, it causes the capillaries in the skin to open up wider and thereby produces the feeling of warmth associated with small dose consumption. Actually the capillaries are letting out heat by dilating thus really cooling the body. Alcohol, like other CNS depressants, lowers body temperature by suppressing the higher regulatory center for body temperature, as well as by vasodilatation.

In the withdrawal syndrome, this pattern is reversed, and fever is associated with other symptoms of withdrawal. These symptoms are: coarse tremors, hallucinations, convulsions, and an acute organic brain syndrome. The entire withdrawal syndrome is called rightly *delirium tremens* or the *D.T.*s. This is so aptly called *delirium tremens* because the most prominent symptoms are delirium, i.e., an acute organic brain syndrome with disorientation, memory impairment, impaired judgment, and intellectual deficits, *and* tremors, very gross shaking of the limbs such that the patient literally could not hold a glass of water and drink from it, plus visual hallucinations. It only occurs where a person is addicted to alcohol, and not merely from an overdose on one occasion.

D.T.s is associated with about a 20% mortality rate despite good treatment. *It is as dangerous to tell an alcoholic on a binge to stop drinking suddenly, as it is to tell a barbiturate addict to stop taking barbiturates suddenly.* In fact, the withdrawal syndromes resemble each other, particularly in the danger of precipitating convulsions if withdrawal is abrupt. It is not even necessary that the alcoholic stop drinking suddenly in order to produce D.T.s. It is known to occur when the alcoholic has merely reduced his intake while continuing to drink. If the alcoholic wants to stop or "dry out" it is best done in a hospital where anticonvulsant medication can be given prophylactically.

ALCOHOL ADDICTION: ALCOHOLISM

How can you tell if a person is addicted to alcohol? If you question him about how he uses alcohol; whether or not he has experienced the "shakes" in the morning or hallucinations (if he doesn't have hallucinations *off* alcohol) while drinking or after stopping drinking, etc. The National Committee on Alcoholism defines major and minor criteria for the diagnosis of alcoholism. The major criteria are associated with the evidence of physical addiction as manifested by the production of withdrawal symptoms (shakes, hallucinations or full blown D.T.s), and the manifestations of alcohol-related disease in the blood, liver, and other organ systems of the body. The major psychological criteria defining psychological dependence are: 1) drinking despite strong medical advice to the contrary; 2) drinking despite known social consequences such as loss of job, loss of spouse, loss of driver's license, etc.; 3) patients subjective evaluation that he has lost control of alcohol consumption.

In addition to the major psychological and physical criteria, there are minor criteria which are *often* associated with alcoholism, but greatly dependent on the peer group habits of the patient. The National Committee on Alcoholism (as printed in the *American Journal* of *Psychiatry*, August 1972) lists the following signs, about which the patient should be questioned, as suggestive of the diagnosis of alcoholism: gulping drinks, drinking in the morning, surrepitious drinking, repeated attempts at abstinence, repeated and multiple medical excuses from work, preference for companions who drink or for bars and taverns, loss of interest in activities not directly associated with drinking, frequent car accidents, frequent changes in residence for poorly defined reasons, outbursts of rage or suicidal gestures while drinking, drinking to relieve anger, insomnia, fatigue, depression or social discomfort and psychological symptoms consistent with permanent organic brain syndrome (see Korsakoff's Psychosis). There are many other *late* criteria but these are the early and middle stage signs of alcoholism.

In general, if you have a good rapport with the patient, he may feel comfortable enough to admit his subjective fears that he has lost control of his alcohol consumption. It is very difficult to correctly diagnose if the patient blatantly denies any of the above signs despite his knowledge to the contrary. Often, none of those signs are acknowledged as present if the patient is a binge drinker or "weekend-alcoholic," i.e., he only gets drunk on weekends or only has the signs during binges which he may or may not admit.

There is another type of drinker, one who is said to have pathological intoxication, for he gets violently drunk or is behaviorally very different after one or two normal size drinks. This type of person may or may not be an alcoholic. Usually the behavior following one or two drinks is extremely different from the person's normal behavior. He may be violent or verbally abusive, he may cry or be suicidal or extremely impulsive. He may also suffer a "blackout;" this also occurs to alcoholics.

Blackouts are periods of total memory loss without the person having been unconscious or drunk necessarily. During the "blackout" many normal or "abnormal" actions may have taken place but all memory for them is lost. They may last for one or two days or possibly longer.

With all of these criteria, which ones should determine whether or not a patient is alcoholic or "merely" on the road to becoming one? The answer lies in asking questions about withdrawal and tolerance phenomena which are *prima facie* evidence of addiction. A person can be alcoholic and never have had D.T.s. Other withdrawal symptoms can be present such as morning "shakes." These shakes occur after someone who has drunk a lot of alcohol (and is addicted to it) sleeps for some time and his blood alcohol level goes down. He awakens with severe shaking of the limbs, almost as gross as the tremors in D.T.s. The usual action taken by the alcoholic is to drink more alcohol to stop the shaking. The "shakes" are probably incipient D.T.s but the symptoms have not yet progressed that far. If a patient admits to getting the shakes in the morning after heavy drinking the evening prior, he should be classified as an alcoholic if he meets at least one major and one minor criteria.

Tolerance is another matter. Some alcoholics will brag about their ability to "hold" their liquor without showing behavioral effects of intoxication. They may also be asked whether they can "hold" their liquor better than most of their peer group and how much can they drink. The consumption of one fifth of a gallon of alcohol daily or for more than one day is evidence of alcoholism. Peer group characteristics can be misleading since the entire peer group can be either alcoholics or incipient alcoholics.

ALCOHOLIC HALLUCINATIONS

Sometimes alcoholics get visual and auditory hallucinations without being psychotic otherwise, and *without* signs of an acute or chronic organic brain syndrome. This is called alcoholic hallucinosis and can occur while drinking or in withdrawal. Here the distinction must be made between an alcoholic schizophrenic and an alcoholic who is hallucinating. History and familiarity with schizophrenic "thought disorders" will sometimes make diagnosis possible. A good question to ask is if the patient has ever experienced hallucinations without alcohol in close temporal proximity to the onset of the hallucinations. (The time period between hallucinations and alcohol consumption should be longer than ten to fourteen days, otherwise the hallucinations can still result from incipient D.T.s.) If the patient hallucinates after a two week absence of alcohol he may be schizophrenic or have another psychosis, or *still* possibly have incipient D.T.s, but this is rather unlikely.

KORSAKOFF'S PSYCHOSIS

This is a variety of *chronic* organic brain syndrome that occurs after very long standing abuse of alcohol. It is rare to see one of the victims of this disease outside a hospital. Korsakoff's psychosis is characterized by the usual signs of organic brain syndrome plus a specific and peculiar type of memory impairment which causes the patient to confabulate. Confabulation is the term used to describe the filling in of memory gaps with plausible sounding (to the patient) stories. For example, if you ask the patient if he has met you before, he may say he has (although in reality he has not) and proceed to give you details of when and where, if you ask him. In general, patients who have memory gaps in other organic brain syndromes will say that they can't remember. Confabulation seems to be almost exclusively confined to this type of alcoholic syndrome. Along with the psychosis there are neurological deficits in the sensation of touch, especially in the lower limbs. This causes the patient to walk peculiarly, by slapping his feet to the ground so he can tell where they are.

To review then for a moment. The major criteria for the diagnosis of alcoholism are divided into two groups; physical and psychological dependence. Evidence of physical dependence is: 1) tolerance; which is defined as being able to ingest enough alcohol to reach a blood level of 150 mg/100 cc *without gross evidence* of *intoxication.* You can estimate this by asking the patient if he seems to be able to drink much more than his peers without getting drunk. If you suspect the peer group to be alcoholic ask how much alcohol he can hold relative to someone whom he knows only drinks occasionally; 2) phenomena such as morning "shakes," hallucinosis, outright D.T.s, and blackouts. Evidence of psychological dependence consists of drinking in the face of strong medical and social constraints and the subjective impression that the patient has lost control of his alcohol consumption.

WHAT TO DO IF YOUR PATIENT IS ALCOHOLIC

Alcoholism is an extraordinarily difficult problem to treat, as is any addiction. Alcohol, like other addicting CNS depressants, can be psychologically depressing. Very often it is a "chicken and egg" problem whether the depression preceded the drinking or vice versa. In my experience the vast majority of alcoholics are depressed. Unfortunately, antidepressants will not solve the problem once the addiction to alcohol has taken hold. Furthermore, antidepressants do not work as well if the person drinks on top of them. Most alcoholics should first be referred to a doctor for a physical checkup and should, as well, be referred to Alcoholics Anonymous. There are very many studies showing that individual psychotherapy is not as effective as AA. If the patient has sufficient psychopathology to warrant individual psychotherapy this should be carried out in conjunction with referral to AA.

CHAPTER XIII

Amine Hypotheses

This chapter is provided for those readers who are interested in a fuller understanding of the current *hypotheses* of drug action. Related to these hypotheses are the following classes of drugs: Antidepressants, lithium, phenothiazines, Reserpine and Alpha-methyl dopa, L-DOPA, and amphetamines. (Note that *sedatives* and *sleeping pills* are *not included*.)

Structural formulas are given for purposes of comparison and need not be memorized.

There are three neurotransmitters presently *hypothesized* to be directly involved with the production of depression, mania, and schizophrenia. These are serotonin, norepinephrine, and dopamine. Serotonin is also known as 5-hydroxytryptamine or 5-HT. Norepinephrine is thought to be more involved with the production of depression or mania, whereas dopamine and 5-HT are thought to be more involved with schizophrenia.

Here are their formulas:

NEUROTRANSMITTERS

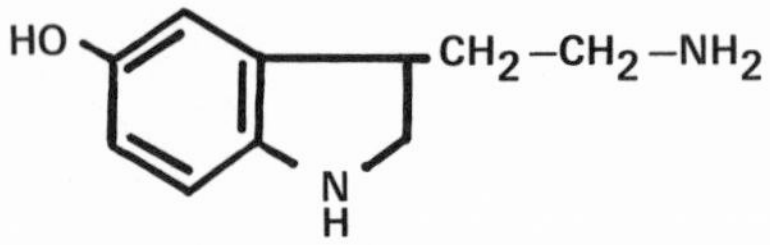

SEROTONIN (5-HT)

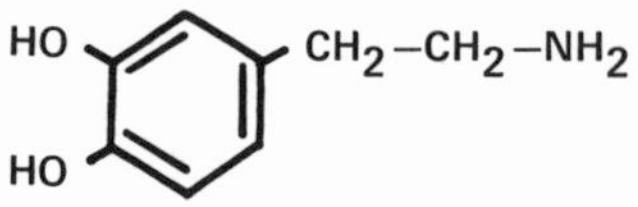

DOPAMINE

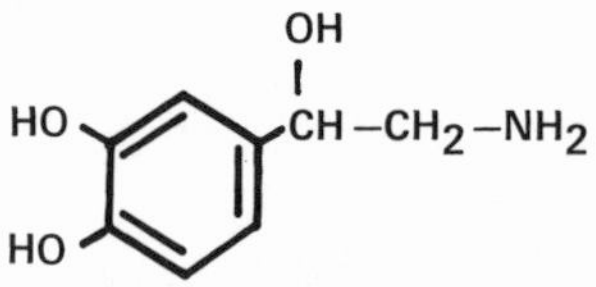

NOREPINEPHRINE

Figure 1

By neurotransmitter is meant that this is a naturally occurring substance in the brain cells and is released by the nerve cell when it is stimulated or fires by itself. It releases the neurotransmitter onto a receptor cell which also may fire and so on, down the line. The neurotransmitters shown in figure 1 are known to exist in groups of cells in specific locations throughout the brain. It is no wonder that these are thought to be associated with psychoses of various types since they look so similar to those drugs which we know are causes of temporary psychoses. Observe the similarities between these neurotransmitters and the drugs shown in figure 2.

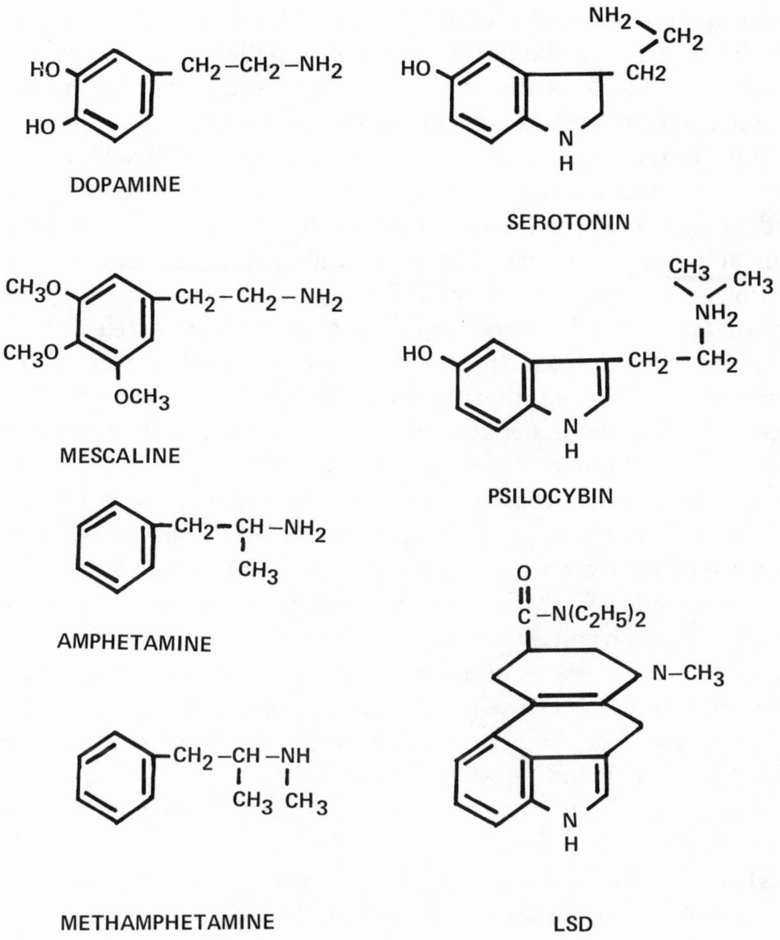

Figure 2

As you will note on the first set of structures, dopamine is also very similar to norepinephrine.

The hypotheses that have been advanced to explain the psychotogenic properties of these drugs is that they in some way mimic the action of the real neurotransmitter on the receptor cell and overstimulate it/or are sufficiently similar to be accepted by the receptor cell, but sufficiently dissimilar enough to cause the reactions we see. There are many investigators still looking for "natural" products of dopamine, norepinephrine or serotonin which the brains or bodies of psychiatric patients produce which would resemble these known psychotomimetic drugs and, hence, perhaps explain why the patient became psychotic.

In order for you to understand the basic mechanisms which are thought to operate in producing drug response, it is necessary to understand the following rather oversimplified principles of nerve cells and their receptors. The nerve cells which have those three neurotransmitters, store them in little granules or vesicles near the end membrane of the nerve cell. When the cell fires it releases the neurotransmitter from the vesicles into the cyptoplasm of the firing cell and from there across the synaptic cleft onto the receptor. The space between the nerve cell and the receptor is known as the synaptic cleft and the whole complex (nerve cell, cleft, and receptor cell) is known as the synapse. Some of the transmitter (in the case of norepinephrine and dopamine) is immediately inactivated in the synaptic cleft by an enzyme known by the abbreviation COMT (catechol-O-methyl transferase). The rest of the neurotransmitter is either inactivated by the MAO (another enzyme, monoamine oxidase) in the receptor cell, or is taken back into the original nerve cell and stored again for future firing (re-uptake). Some of the neurotransmitter is also inactivated by the MAO in the original nerve cell, both after it is released from the granules and after it is taken back (re-uptaken) by the cell. Figure 3 should aid visualization of the action.

There are several drugs which work by preventing or enhancing the re-uptake mechanism of the original firing cell. Other drugs deplete the granules of their supply, and other drugs prevent the action of MAO and thereby increase the supply of neurotransmitter within the nerve cell. All three neurotransmitters are known chemically as monoamines, that is they have *one* amine (NH_2) group on them. There are other neurotransmitters which are not monoamines but we need not be concerned about them here.

One hypothesis states, very concisely, and very roughly that increased amounts of norepinephrine in certain nerve cells or

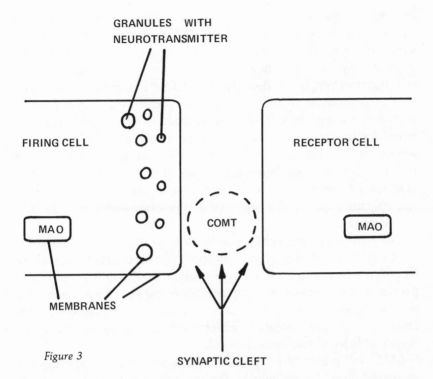

GRANULES   WITH
NEUROTRANSMITTER

FIRING CELL

RECEPTOR CELL

MAO

COMT

MAO

MEMBRANES

Figure 3

SYNAPTIC CLEFT

endings and ultimately, therefore, on the receptor cells will cause excitability and lead to mania. Decreased amounts of norepinephrine however, will conversely lead to depression.

Another hypothesis concerning schizophrenia relates dopamine-containing neurons to schizophrenia because it is known that antipsychotic drugs produce "Parkinsonian" symptoms, always and inseparably (so far) from the antipsychotic agents' effects. Since it *is* known that Parkinson's Disease *results* from problems in the dopamine-containing neurons, they reason that antipsychotic drugs must also act upon not only *those* neurons producing Parkinsonian symptoms, but also those neurons involved in the psychosis.

DRUG ACTIONS: HYPOTHESES

Let us begin with those drugs which we know are antidepressants, either temporary (amphetamines) or more prolonged (tricyclics). As you can see by the structure of amphetamine it closely resembles both dopamine and norepinephrine. There is some thought that it produces excitement, good mood, and euphoria by acting as if it were norepinephrine on the receptor cell; it, however, is not destroyed by COMT in the synaptic cleft. It is also thought to release both norepinephrine and dopamine from the storage vesicles *and* to slightly inhibit MAO, this terminating the action of both norepinephrine and dopamine. No wonder it is a *stimulant*. Since it resembles dopamine so closely, it is also thought possible that it overstimulates the dopamine neurons in the same way as it causes overstimulation of norepinephrine neurons (by mimicry and release) and hence can lead to psychosis.

Tricyclics have been shown to inhibit the re-uptake mechanism, which is the most important way that cells terminate the action of the released neurotransmitter. Tricyclics are thought primarily to prevent the re-uptake of norepinephrine and thus leave more of it on the receptor cell. This more continuous stimulation of the receptor by the released norepinephrine is thought to be responsible for the increased mood.

MAO inhibitors, it is hypothesized, also can be responsible for increased mood by preventing the degradation and inactivation of the norepinephrine, thus leaving more of it both inside the firing cell and on the receptor cell.

As was noted, both tricyclics and MAO inhibitors take about two weeks to start working *behaviorally* or in terms of subjective mood. It is not clear yet why this is so. Lithium on the other side, being an antimanic drug, is thought to *enhance* the re-uptake mechanism and prevent release of the neurotransmitter, norepinephrine, by doing something to the limiting membrane of the firing cell. Just how lithium can also work as an antidepressant in some manic-depressives is not clear from this explanation, in fact it should not be possible. Investigation has yet to clarify this paradox. Phenothiazines can cause the symptoms of dopamine *deficiency* which are called "Parkinsonian" symptoms, because persons with Parkinson's Disease are *known* to have a dopamine deficiency in certain areas of the brain. These areas are NOT responsible for the psychiatric symptomatology. However, because it is thought that phenothiazines must block the dopamine in these areas in order to produce "Parkinsonian" symptoms, they must also block the *dopamine neurons* in the areas which *are* responsible for psychotic psychiatric symptoms. The question is rightly asked therefore, "How come not all patients on phenothiazines get "Parkinsonian" side effects?" The answer lies probably in the dose and response curve of the entire population. Probably every patient taking phenothiazines would develop "Parkinsonian" side effects if the dose was high enough. Luckily, about 80% of patients treated have an antipsychotic effect from phenothiazines *without* having "Parkinsonian" side effects. This must say something about the sensitivity of the various receptors involved. In fact, some recent evidence indicates that there *are* two types of dopamine receptor-neurons (Klawans, 1973).

A word about L-DOPA. L-DOPA is given to patients with Parkinson's Disease to increase the amount of dopamine at the deficient sites in the brain. As you might expect, about 10% of the patients so treated get psychiatric symptomatology, ranging from psychosis to mania to depression. Psychosis might be easy to understand, given the above explanations. However, mania is also easily understandable if you know that dopamine can be converted to norepinephrine very easily, and it is excess norepinephrine which is thought to be responsible for mania. In the same way, drugs which block the conversion from dopamine to norepinephrine might be responsible for depression. Or further, drugs which resemble dopamine sufficiently to be converted to the norepinephrine-like compound might cause depression if they block the real norepinephrine. Such a drug is the common antihypertensive agent alpha-methyl dopa (tradename: Aldomet). Aldomet can and does cause depression in about 5-10% of persons treated with it who are evidently predisposed to depression to begin with. That predisposition is probably biological, but this is still hotly debated.

Reserpine, another antihypertensive drug, also causes severe depression in about 10% of those patients treated with it. It is known to deplete the norepinephrine storage granules of their supply of norepinephrine and this presumably leads to depression. Again, querying why all persons treated do not get depressed, accents the incompleteness of our knowledge in this field.

REFERENCES

Detre, T.P. and Jarecki, H.G. *Modern Psychiatric Treatment*, Lippincott, Philadelphia, Pa., 1971.

Freedman, A.M. and Kaplan, H.J. *Comprehensive Textbook of Psychiatry*, Williams & Wilkins, Baltimore, Md., 1967.

Harrison, T.R., et al. (Eds.). *Principles of Internal Medicine*, McGraw-Hill, New York, 1974.

Klawans, H.L., Jr., "Pharmacology of Tardive Dyskinesis," *Amer. J. Psychiat. 130*:1 (January 1973).

Klein, D.F. and Davis, J.M. *Diagnosis and Drug Treatment of Psychiatric Disorders*, Williams & Wilkins, Baltimore, Md., 1969.

Lebensohm, Z.M. and Jenkins, R.B. "Improvement of Parkinsonism in depressed patients treated with ECT," *Amer. J. Psychiat. 132*:3(March 1975).

National Commission on Marijuana and Drug Abuse. *"Marajuana, a Signal of Misunderstanding*, New American Library, New York, 1972.

Modern Psychiatric Treatment Detre, T.P. & Jarecki, H.G., Lippincott 1971.

Diagnosis and Drug Treatment of Psychiatric Disorders Klein, D.F.; Davis, J.M., Williams & Wilkins 1969.

Psychotropic Drug Side Effects Shader, R.I. & DiMascio, A., Williams & Wilkins 1970.

Comprehensive Textbook of Psychiatry Freedman, A.M. & Kaplan, H.J., Williams & Wilkins 1967.

Principles of Internal Medicine Harrison, T.R. Ed. Wintrobe M.M., et al. McGraw Hill 1974.

National Commission on Marijuana and Drug Abuse, "Marajuana, a Signal of Misunderstanding, The New American Library, New York, 1972.

Klawans, H.L., Jr., Pharmacology of Tardive Dyskinesis, Amer. J. Psychiat. 130:1 (January 1973).

Lebensohn, Z.M. and Jenkins, R.B. "Improvement of Parkinsonism in depressed patients treated with ECT," Amer. J. Psychiat. 132:3(March 1975).

Shader and Dimascio, Psychotropic Drug Side Effects, Williams & Wilkins, 1970.

ACETYLCHOLINE: A known neuro-transmitter in the peripheral nervous system and neurotransmitter of the parasympathetic nervous system which is a subgroup of peripheral nerves. Also hypothesized to be neurotransmitter in central nervous system.

AKATHISIA: A side effect of pheno-thiazines *and other* antipsychotic drugs: it is the subjective sensation of not being able to sit still; of having to move legs and feet particularly.

ANALGESIC: Pain relieving.

ANERGIA: Lack of energy.

ANGINA PECTORIS: A syndrome char-acterized by pain in the chest around the heart, occasionally profuse sweat-ing and anxiety. It is usually associ-ated with a real temporary deficit in blood supply to the heart muscle causing severe pain which often can be relieved by nitroglycerin tablets under the tongue.

ANOREXIA: Loss of appetite.

ANTICHOLINERGIC: Having properties which interfere with the functioning

of the cholinergic (in most cases para-sympathetic) nervous system.

BIPOLAR: In this text bipolar refers to persons with manic-depressive illness in either phase of that illness or having a history compatible with such a diagnosis.

CHOLINERGIC: Refers to nervous systems utilizing acetylcholine as their neurotransmitter—in this text pri-marily the parasympathetic nervous system.

CONFABULATION: A peculiar way of filling in gaps in memory by making up plausible-sounding but false stories; primarily seen in alcoholic brain disease.

CNS: Central nervous system: the brain and spinal cord.

CYCLOTHYMIC: Refers to type of personality in which the person tends to have mild depressions and mild elations as distinguished from manic-depressive illness where the mood swings are much more intense.

CNS DEPRESSANT: A drug which causes slowing or decrease in excitability of nerve cells in the CNS: all sleeping pills, narcotics, tranquilizers, and alcohol are CNS depressants.

DELUSION: A belief held by a person *which is not culturally* accepted and which cannot be changed by reasoning; a false belief.

EEG (electroencephalograph) Commonly known as brain wave test. A form of polygraph specifically designed to pick up frequencies of electromagnetic waves emitted by the brain.

EPINEPHRINE: A substance released by the adrenal gland which causes signs of sympathetic reaction.

HALLUCINATION: A sensory perception which has no basis in reality; may be visual, auditory, olfactory (smell) etc.

HYPERSOMNIA: Excessive sleeping —more than eight hours per night in an adult.

HYPERVENTILATION: Excessive breathing—usually too deep for too long a period of time; a syndrome consisting of numbness and tingling of the fingertips and toes bilaterally, chest pain and anxiety, due to overbreathing.

HYPNOTIC: Sleep producing—the medical term for sleep-producing drugs. drugs.

HYPOGLYCEMIA: Low blood sugar.

HYPOMANIA: A state of increased motor activity, excessively good mood; *not* psychotic, necessarily.

HYSTERICAL, HYSTERIA: Terms used to denote a neurotic condition wherein the person converts anxiety into physical symptoms and sometimes mental symptoms such as hysterical amnesia. The physical symptoms are varied but can be paralysis of a limb, blindness, etc. These physical or mental symptoms do not usually follow known anatomic pathways and can be removed under pentobarbital or hypnosis.

I.M.: Intramuscularly—refers to how a medicine is injected into a muscle.

ILLUSION: An incorrect sensory perception having some basis in reality as opposed to a hallucination. It is an illusion for example when the road looks wet in front of you because of the angle of the sun on it, when it is really dry.

ISCHEMIA: Insufficient blood supply.

MAOI: Monoamine oxidase inhibitor— type of antidepressant.

MANIA: A state of extreme increase in motor activity, verbal activity and euphoric or hostile mood; generally reserved for these symptoms in combination with psychosis.

MENTATION: Thinking or thought processes.

NARCOTIC: Producing numbness; usually also produce sleep or lethargy in moderate doses. Medically used as pain relievers.

NEURON: Nerve cell.

NOREPINEPHRINE: A neurotransmitter in the CNS and peripheral sympathetic nervous system.

OBS: Organic brain syndrome—deficits in memory and other intellectual functions due to disease or dysfunction of the neurons in the brain.

ORTHOSTATIC HYPOTENSION: Temporary decrease in blood pressure when person changes positions from sitting or lying down to standing. The person feels dizzy temporarily but returns to normal in a few seconds.

Generally a side effect of major tranquilizers and antidepressants.

PARASYMPATHETIC, NERVOUS
SYSTEM: A part of peripheral
nervous system concerned with vegetative functions.

PARESTHESIA: Numbness and tingling of
the extremities—example when foot
"falls asleep".

PATHOLOGIC INTOXICATION: A
person who gets drunk with blackouts
and possibly violent on one or two
normal drinks.

PERISTALSIS: Consecutive constriction
of intestinal segments pushing food
along.

PHENOTHIAZINE: A major tranquilizing
drug as opposed to minor tranquilizers.

PHYSIOLOGICAL: Refers to the process
of the functioning of various *body*
systems.

REM: Rapid eye movement stage of sleep.

SEDATIVE: Calming, quieting—a drug
causing decrease in nervous excitement.

SOMATIC: Refers to the body as opposed
to psychic referring to the mind.

SYMPATHETIC NERVOUS SYSTEM:
Part of the peripheral nervous system
as well as certain connections in the
CNS—responsible for "fight or flight"
reactions and general body homeo-
stasis.

TOLERANCE: The physiological process
whereby the user of a drug can tolerate physically more drug than is usual
to produce the desired effect.
Tolerance implies the need to increase
the dose of a drug in order to keep ob-
taining the desired response. Cross

tolerance occurs when drugs with
similar effects produce tolerance to all
those drugs with similar effects, e.g.,
if a person is tolerant to barbiturates
he may also be tolerant to nonbarbiturate sleeping pills.

TOXIC: Poisonous; a state of mind or
body resulting from poisonous drug
or excessive dosage of medicines or
endogenous toxins.

TREMOR: Fine or coarse shaking of limbs,
generally hands.

TRICYCLIC: A type of antidepressant.

UNCINATE FITS: Another synonym for
psychomotor epilepsy or temporal
lobe epilepsy. In this condition the
patient has violent outbursts of rage
which last a few minutes to hours.

UNIPOLAR: In this text refers to a type of
depression generally formerly called
endogenous depression, characterized
by weight loss, sleep loss, and
agitation.

Glossary of Drugs

Generic Name	Brand	Company
	Major Tranquilizers **(Antipsychotic Agents)**	
Phenothiazines		
Acetophenazine	Tindal	Schering
Butaperazine	Repoise	Robins
Carphenazine	Proketazine	Wyeth
Chlorpromazine	Thorazine	Smith, Kline & French
Dixyrazine	Esucos	Union Chimiques Belge*
Fluphenazine	Prolixin, Permitil	Squibb, White
Mesoridazine	Serentil	Boehringer Ingelheim
Methotrimeprazine	Levoprome	Lederle
Perphenazine	Trilafon	Schering
Piperacetazine	Quide	Dow Pharmaceutical
Prochlorperazine	Compazine	Smith, Kline & French
Promazine	Sparine	Wyeth
Propericiazine	Neuleptil	Rhone-Poulenc*
Thiazinamium	Multergan	Rhone-Poulenc*
Thiethylperazine	Torecan	Boehringer Ingleheim
Thioproperazine	Majeptil	Rhone-Poulenc*
Thioridazine	Mellaril	Sandoz
Trifluoperazine	Stelazine	Smith, Kline & French
Triflupromazine	Vesprin	Squibb
Butyrophenones		
Dehydrobenzperidol	Innovar	McNeil
Haloperidol	Haldol	McNeil
Thioxanthenes		
Chlorprothixene	Taractan	Roche
Thiothixene	Navane	Pfizer Roerig
Reserpines		
Deserpidine	Harmonyl	Abbott
Rescinnamine	Moderil	Pfizer
Reserpine	Serpasil and others	Ciba and others
	Antidepressants	
Tricyclics		
Amitriptyline	Elavil	Merck
Desipramine	Pertofrane, Norpramin	USV Pharmaceitucal Geigy, Lakeside

Glossary of Drugs (cont.)

Generic Name	Brand	Company
Imipramine	Tofranil	Geigy
Nortriptyline	Aventyl	Lilly
Protriptyline	Vivactil	Merck
Trimipramine	Surmontil	Rhone-Poulenc

MAO Inhibitors

Etryptamine	Monase (withdrawn)	Upjohn
Iproniazid	Marsilid (withdrawn)	Roche
Isocarboxazid	Marplan	Roche
Mebanazine	Actomol	Imperial Chemical Industry
Pargyline	Eutonyl	Abbott
Phenelzine	Nardil	Warner
Pheniprazine	Catron (withdrawn)	Lakeside
Tranylcypromine	Parnate	Smith, Kline & French

Prescribable Stimulants

Amphetamine	Benzedrine	Smith, Kline & French
Dextro-Amphetamine	Dexedrine	Smith, Kline & French
Deanol	Deaner	Riker
Methamphetamine	Desoxyn	Abbott
Methylphenidate	Ritalin	Ciba

Nonbarbiturate Minor Tranquilizers and Sedatives

Chlordiazepoxide	Librium	Roche
Chlormethazanone	Trancopal	Sterling-Winthrop
Diazepam	Valium	Roche
Hydroxyzine	Vistaril, Atarax	Pfizer, Roerig
Meprobamate	Miltown, Equanil	Wallace, Wyeth
Oxazepam	Serax	Wyeth

Nonbarbiturate Sleeping Pills (Hypnotics)

Ethchlorvynol	Placidyl	Abbott
Ethinamate	Valmid	Dista
Flurazepam	Dalmane	Roche
Glutethimide	Doriden	Ciba, USV Pharmaceutical
Methaqualone	Quaalude	Rorer
Methyprylon	Noludar	Roche

Subject Index